NO MORE
HEADACHES
NO MORE
MIGRAINES

Zuzana Bic, DrPH
L. Francis Bic, PhD

AVERY PUBLISHING GROUP

Garden City Park • New York

The information and advice contained in this book are based upon the research and the personal and professional experiences of the authors. They are not intended as a substitute for consulting with your physician or other health care provider. The publisher and authors are not responsible for any adverse effects or consequences resulting from the use of any of the suggestions or procedures discussed in this book. All matters pertaining to your physical health should be supervised by a health care professional. It is a sign of wisdom, not cowardice, to seek a second or third opinion.

Cover Design: Eric Macaluso
Typesetter: Richard Morrock
Editor: Joan Taber Altieri

Avery Publishing Group
120 Old Broadway
Garden City Park, New York 11040
1–800–548–5757
www.averypublishing.com

Cataloging-in-Publication Data

Bic, Zuzana.
    No more headaches, no more migraines / Zuzana
Bic, L. Francis Bic. — 1st ed.
    p. cm.
    Includes bibliographical references and index.
    ISBN: 0-89529-924-0

    1. Headache—Prevention—Popular works.
    2. Migraine—Prevention—Popular works.
    I. Bic, L. Francis. II. Title.

RC392.B53 1999   616'.8'491
                                                 QBI99-994

Printed in the United States of America

10   9   8   7   6   5   4   3   2   1

Contents

This book is dedicated to our son Alexander.

Acknowledgments

Many people played a role in bringing this book to completion, and our gratitude to them is greater than we can express. We are grateful to the staff at Avery Publishing, particularly the publisher Rudy Shur for choosing this book for publication, and to Joan Altieri and Joanne Abrams for guiding it from its earliest draft stages to completion.

Much of this book is based on research conducted at Loma Linda University's School of Public Health, and it involved a number of individuals who contributed their time and effort. Dr. Glen G. Blix and Dr. Helen P. Hopp provided guidance, stimulating discussions, and constant encouragement throughout the entire project, which greatly advanced its progress. Dr. Michael J. Schell of the University of North Carolina, Chapel Hill invested many hours of patient instruction and advice in statistical analysis. Dr. Frances M. Leslie of the University of California, Irvine provided valuable insights and organizational help for conducting the research.

The work also involved a number of individuals at other institutions. Dr. Wes Youngberg was very supportive of the initial research ideas on headache, and it was at his Preventive Care & Lifestyle Medicine practice that the connection between type II diabetes and headache was first observed. Dr. Eva E. Katz, from Family Medicine Practice, Irvine, provided the space in her medical practice and referred many of her patients to the study. Patricia B. Collette-Penzo and Sandhya R. Upasani contributed to the project in a number of important ways. Marlene E. Strauss helped with the writing and editing of the first draft of this book.

We are indebted to all the above individuals, without whose dedication this project would not have been possible. We would also like to express our sincere appreciation to all the headache sufferers who participated in the headache research study. Their spirit of volunteerism made it possible to pioneer a new approach to headache treatment.

Finally, our greatest gratitude belongs to our parents, Ludmila Strakova and Lubomir and Olga Bic, for their boundless trust, support, and encouragement.

Preface

No More Headaches, No More Migraines is a practical self-help guide to managing headaches that is based on a research study I conducted at Loma Linda University's School of Public Health and on my clinical experience with headache patients. It presents a new approach, called *lifestyle modification*, to treating headaches involving preventive care, or *lifestyle medicine*.

I was trained in conventional medicine and neurology, and I have always been a staunch supporter of prevention. But rather than pursue a career as a practitioner of traditional Western medicine, I have dedicated my work to the principle that the best way to cure a disease is to prevent it. I believe that many chronic diseases can be alleviated or even completely reversed by using lifestyle modification treatments. This conviction led me to Loma Linda University, a school renowned for its pioneering contributions to medical science, where I obtained a second doctorate, in public health, and became a specialist in preventive care.

I have devoted almost six years to studying the widespread and elusive problem of headaches. Very few people do not suffer from occasional headaches, and many experience them on a weekly or daily basis. Where do they come from? What are their main causes? Is it stress, certain types of foods, too much work, lack of sleep, lack of exercise, caffeine, alcohol, nicotine? Or is it simply a genetic defect we can do little about? What intrigued me about the headache problem was the very wide range of seemingly unrelated factors that can trigger many types of headaches. I theorized that if there were common biochemical imbalances linking the various factors, there must be a uniform treatment for headaches. One of the most important headache triggers turned out to be levels of fat—*lipids* and *fatty acids*—in the blood. Fat levels in the body are affected by the same things that can trigger headaches, including lack of physical activity, emotional upset, inadequate sleep, stress, certain types of foods, and poorly balanced nutrition. This led me to conduct a clinical study that explored the nutrition of patients suffering from migraine headaches. However, instead of focusing on specific types of foods, I introduced my headache patients to a balanced program of nutrition, which they followed for a period of several weeks. The result was a dramatic decrease in the frequency, severity, and duration of their headaches. And in many cases, the headaches disappeared completely.

After publishing my results, I began to use the nutrition approach in my clinical practice. I also expanded the lifestyle modification treatment to include other essential components—especially physical activity and stress management. After years of working with patients suffering from headaches and other chronic diseases, I began to realize that one of the greatest challenges in preventive care and lifestyle medicine is to convince patients to take charge of their own health. This generally requires a shift in the patient's lifestyle. Most people know very well what it means to have a healthy lifestyle; but knowing what should be done and doing it are two very different things. To achieve and sustain significant lifestyle modification requires specific strategies that bring about changes gradually. It is my hope that the techniques of lifestyle modification, which I have developed from practical experience, will help headache sufferers throughout the world.

Dr. Zuzana Bic

Introduction

Few people have not suffered from headaches. In fact, headaches have been a common ailment throughout the history of humankind. Healthcare practitioners have experimented with a remarkably broad range of headache treatments, including spiritual or ritualistic healing, acupuncture, herbal remedies, synthetic drugs, and surgery; but the problem persists. Even modern medicine has not been able to offer a solution to the problem of headaches. The best it can do is provide patients with pain relievers to alleviate their immediate suffering. Unfortunately, many drugs, especially when they are taken over an extended period, produce various side effects, some of which can be serious. Most of you will probably agree that frequent use of such drugs is not a sensible, long-term solution.

Perhaps even more important, headaches are usually the result of another health- or lifestyle-related problem. The famous sociologist Norman Cousins once said, "The best way to eliminate [pain] is to eliminate the abuses—tension, stress, worry, idleness, boredom, frustration, suppressed rage, insufficient sleep, overeating, poorly balanced diet, smoking, excessive drinking, inadequate exercise, stale air, or any of the other abuses encountered by the human body in modern society." His remark captures the essence of this book. While most headache remedies focus on eliminating headaches after they have occurred, this book focuses on their *prevention*. Once a headache is already in progress, it is too late. The only thing you can do is try to relieve the pain. A far better approach is to avoid or remove the conditions that cause headaches.

The solution—which we call the *lifestyle modification approach*—is a treatment based on the results of a study I conducted at Loma Linda University, a leading institution in preventive medicine. One of the most important outcomes of this study was the development of a new theory for understanding the biochemical processes involved in headaches and their relationship with various lifestyle factors. I tried the lifestyle modification approach on a group of patients diagnosed with chronic migraines. The outcome was a dramatic decrease in the frequency, intensity, and duration of headaches in over 90 percent of my patients. This, in turn, resulted in a significant decrease in their use of medication. And in many cases, patients' headaches disappeared completely.

The results of my study were published in scientific literature, which received national attention and generated a flurry of headlines in the general press. Even national magazines such as *Prevention, Better Homes and Gardens, The Ladies' Home Journal, Men's Health,* and *Glamour* featured the Loma Linda study and offered advice to headache sufferers. These articles were extremely important in alerting people to the lifestyle modification approach, but they were too brief to be of practical value to headache sufferers. This book provides a comprehensive collection of materials; it explains the findings of the study and offers practical advice about how to alleviate chronic headaches. *No More Head-*

aches, No More Migraines is an extension of my clinical practice; and it gives me a way to share my knowledge and experience with thousands of headache sufferers who are beyond the scope of my practice. It provides specific techniques and strategies that can easily be incorporated into your busy daily routine and that are likely to bring about the gradual lifestyle changes necessary to reverse your headache problem.

The Loma Linda study and the resulting clinical experience with headache patients distinguished three specific areas of lifestyle modification. The first and most important is a balanced, nutritional diet that is low in fat and refined sugar and high in complex carbohydrates. However, unlike many other nutrition-based approaches to headache treatment, this book does not advocate *elimination diets* that forbid the consumption of certain types of foods or nutrients. Rather, it will teach you specific techniques and strategies to achieve a gradual change in your dietary preferences, leading to a voluntary shift toward healthier nutrition, with no feelings of deprivation.

The second area of lifestyle modification is physical activity. The book will explain how a sedentary lifestyle can cause headaches, and it will show you how to improve your physical well-being. The techniques are designed to introduce additional physical tasks and exercises gradually, without requiring strong willpower.

The third area of lifestyle modification is devoted to understanding the negative long-term effects of stress on your health. The most important realization is that stress is often a matter of perception. While you may not be able to eliminate the things that trigger stress, there are techniques you can employ that will reduce the impact of stress triggers. These techniques can also improve sleep patterns, which has been shown to be an important factor in controlling headaches.

In addition, we will look beyond the headache problem by considering other chronic diseases such as hypertension, diabetes, coronary heart disease, and even cancer. Very few headaches are the direct result of an existing acute condition. In fact, in most instances, there is no detectable physiological cause, and only the symptoms of headache are treated. Nevertheless, recurring headaches are often the result of a larger problem, which may be caused by a multitude of lifestyle factors. If these problems are ignored, your body's natural defense mechanisms may become exhausted, which would leave you susceptible to another, seemingly unrelated, chronic disease. By finding and eliminating the causes of headaches, you will improve your immediate quality of life and you will fight an important battle against much more serious conditions that could await you many years down the road.

No More Headaches, No More Migraines will guide you through a brief history of headaches to a future that may leave you headache-free. Chapter 1 provides the necessary background with a brief historical perspective on the headache problem. It points out the shortcomings of existing treatments and explains the classification of headaches accepted by the World Health Organization and the International Headache Society.

Chapter 2, which is based on my Loma Linda study, describes the various biochemical imbalances in the body that have been linked to headaches. It also identifies the lifestyle factors that may cause these imbalances to occur. This information points to the need for new treatments based on specific lifestyle modifications to reverse negative factors and prevent headaches from occurring.

The next three chapters make up the core of this book, each focusing on one major area of lifestyle associated with headaches. Chapter 3 considers nutrition and the closely related subject of taste, which is often thought to be in direct conflict with the concept of a healthy diet. This chapter shows that it is possible to modify your sense of taste and adopt a different style of eating. It provides practical techniques and strategies to achieve a gradual shift toward more balanced eating, without feeling deprived and without the need for strong self-discipline.

Chapter 4 focuses on physical activity and exercise in general. Exercise that is perceived as a punishment can't possibly be effective. Instead, it is necessary to develop a liking for a certain level of physical activity. This chapter presents strategies and techniques to increase physical activity, which you can easily incorporate into your busy life.

Chapter 5 discusses stress, which is directly linked to headaches. Eliminating stress-producing events or situations is often difficult, but there are effective ways to train our minds and perceptions to minimize the impact of stress on body chemistry. Like the previous two chapters, this chapter presents specific suggestions about managing stress to prevent the recurrence of headache.

Given that all lifestyle changes must be introduced gradually, it is often difficult to assess the effectiveness of the strategies. Chapter 6 introduces ways of measuring your progress at home without special training. You can keep track of your progress by recording the measurements in journals.

At the end of these chapters, you will find the appendices. Appendix A lists the nutritional contents of many important foods, and Appendix B provides a helpful reading list for readers who want to learn more.

No More Headaches, No More Migraines looks at the headache problem from a fresh, new perspective and does not try to isolate or correct individual imbalances artificially. If you suffer from headaches or you want to help someone else who does, this book offers solutions that really work. The techniques have been proven time and time again. You have nothing to lose by trying them—except your headaches.

CHAPTER 1

Headaches and Their Remedies

Lord, how my head aches!
What a head have I!
It beats as it would fall
In twenty pieces.

—William Shakespeare

A s far as anyone knows, headaches have plagued humankind since prerecorded history; and despite centuries of pain and decades of scientific research, people continue to suffer. As you will see, there are many types of headaches and all sorts of remedies from prescription and over-the-counter medications to alternative approaches such as meditation and exercise. This chapter discusses the various classifications of headaches, their history, and their most common treatments.

CLASSIFICATION OF HEADACHES

If you are a headache sufferer, you have probably heard a number of terms that describe different types of headaches. The most commonly used terms are migraines, tension headaches, cluster headaches, mixed headaches, sinus headaches, menstrual headaches, primary headaches, secondary headaches, and chronic headaches. These terms are very clear and easy to understand. But confusion can arise because most headaches don't fit neatly into one specific category. There are also many myths, so much anecdotal data, and sometimes outright incorrect information about headaches. Furthermore, books don't always use the same classifications, and physicians rarely have the time to explain the complete picture to their patients.

There is an official classification of headaches and related disorders that has been accepted by the World Health Organization and is the basis of all conventional headache treatments. The classification distinguishes thirteen headache categories, each of which is subdivided into more specific categories and subcategories. While the details of this classification are exhaustive, the vast majority of headaches fall into only a few categories. The sections that follow will concentrate on the types of headaches that are most likely to respond to the lifestyle modification approach presented in this book.

Even if you have been diagnosed with a specific type of headache and are certain of its origins, you may still want to read this section. Why? Some headaches are the direct result of another disorder, such as hypertension or diabetes. You will find that the lifestyle modification approach to the elimination of headaches is not restricted to curing headaches. In fact, lifestyle modification can improve or even completely reverse other chronic illnesses such as hypertension, hyperlipidemia, and diabetes. By improving medical conditions such as these, the associated headaches are also likely to be relieved.

The international headache classification was developed and published in 1988 by the Headache Classification Committee of the International Headache Society. Since that time, it has been translated into many languages and is used worldwide to diagnose and treat headaches. The classification categorizes *primary* and *secondary* headaches. As the name implies, primary headaches are not associated with any other disease or organic disorder. They include migraines, tension headaches, cluster headaches, and a variety of miscellaneous headaches. On the other hand, secondary headaches are the result of some other medical problem. Although secondary headaches account for only 10 percent of headaches, there are hundreds of possible causes—head injuries, blood vessel disorders, viral and bacterial infections, metabolic and neurological ailments, and various diseases of the neck, eyes, ears, nose, and teeth. Other causes may include the use or elimination of certain foods or chemical substances, such as alcohol, nicotine, pain relievers, and oral contraceptives.

Although primary headaches are the most common type of headaches, they are difficult to treat using conventional medical approaches because their triggers and their symptoms vary widely. The following sections examine the main characteristics of primary headaches.

Migraine Headaches

The international headache classification identifies several different types of migraines, the most important of which are *migraine without aura*—also called common migraine— and *migraine with aura*—or classic migraine. Researchers have conducted dozens of studies on migraines, and most conclude that women suffer from migraines more frequently than do men. Migraine without aura has the following characteristics:

- The attack commonly lasts between 4 and 72 hours and can occur any time of day or night.

- The pain is throbbing or pulsating and is generally *unilateral*—on one side of the head.

- The headache is moderate to severe in intensity, which means it inhibits or prohibits daily activities.

- The headache is exacerbated by routine physical activity, such as walking.

- The headache is accompanied by nausea and/or vomiting.

- Sufferers are hypersensitive to light and/or noise.

Migraine with aura has the same general characteristics as those listed above, but it is accompanied by an aura. The most common form of aura is a visual disturbance that distorts the normal field of vision. Some patients remark that they seem to be looking through shimmering hot air rising from a fire or stove. Other forms of aura may include numbness and difficulty speaking. An aura usually precedes the pain by less than one hour.

Tension Headaches

Almost everyone has experienced tension headaches, which are the most common and least severe headaches. Tension headaches also seem to affect women more frequently than they do men. The classification distinguishes between *episodic*, or occasional tension headaches, and *chronic*, or regular, tension headaches. Tension headaches have the following characteristics:

- The attacks may last anywhere from 30 minutes to several days.

- The pain seems to press or tighten against the head, and it is generally *bilateral*—on both sides of the head.

- The intensity of the pain is mild to moderate, permitting the person to continue work and other daily activities.

- The pain does not increase with physical activity.

- The headache is sometimes accompanied by muscle tenderness, but rarely by other side effects.

Cluster Headaches

Cluster headaches are less common than migraines or tension headaches, but they produce the most severe pain. Unlike other types of headaches, cluster headaches seem to afflict more men than women. They generally start to occur in people in their late twenties. The most common characteristics of cluster headaches are the following:

- The attacks are brief, lasting between fifteen minutes and a few hours, but they occur in "clusters"—from once every other day to several times a day for several weeks or longer.

- The pain is generally centered around or behind one eye or temple and is very severe. It can cause a high level of agitation and desperation.

- The headaches are sometimes accompanied by tearing, nasal congestion, or sweating, but rarely by nausea, vomiting, or increased sensitivity to light or noise.

A BRIEF HISTORY OF HEADACHES

Headaches are a common intrusion in our lives, and we tend to blame our hectic modern lifestyles for this recurrent ailment. But when we look at the history of headaches, we see that the problem has persisted for thousands of years. The reason is that the lifestyle factors that cause headache suffering—improperly balanced nutrition, lack of physical activity, and stress—may have their origins in the dawn of human civilization.

The earliest indications that headaches may be an ancient problem date back to prerecorded history. Archaeologists have found centuries-old skulls that have markings similar to those produced by *trepanation*—an ancient procedure that involves drilling or cutting a small hole into the skull in order to relieve headaches. Surprisingly, many

Headaches as Early Warning Signals

Pain is one of our most important protective mechanisms because it is a warning signal that some part of the body is injured. We automatically try to avoid pain. For example, a child who touches something hot will usually learn not to touch that thing again. But headaches produce pain whose origins are not immediately obvious. We don't always know what triggers headache pain, so it is impossible to discover how to prevent it from occurring again. Recurrent headaches are a signal that you are suffering from physiological imbalances, and these imbalances are usually the result of lifestyle factors.

Headaches occur most frequently and with the greatest severity in people under the age of forty-five. It is interesting that as incidences of headaches begin to diminish with advancing age, many chronic diseases begin to become apparent. Since the various lifestyle factors that cause headaches are the same as those that cause many chronic diseases, headaches can be seen as early warning signs of possible future diseases. Therefore, it is logical to conclude that appropriate lifestyle changes will reduce the immediate suffering produced by headaches and will greatly reduce the risk of developing other problems in the future.

The next few pages discuss some examples of the most common chronic diseases that may be caused by lifestyle factors, including lack of physical activity, excessive stress, smoking, immoderate consumption of alcohol or caffeine, and improperly balanced diets. Repeated headaches indicate the presence of some or all of these factors and thus an increased risk for developing these diseases.

Type II Diabetes and Other Insulin-Related Disorders

Type II diabetes is a disease that impairs the body's ability to use or produce insulin. Other disorders involving insulin include hyperinsulinemia and insulin resistance. Doctors generally recommend a diet low in fat and refined sugar for patients with these disorders. Thus, the same nutritional modifications recommended for headache prevention will also reverse these insulin-related disorders or prevent them from developing later in life.

Cardiovascular Diseases

The development of chronic cardiovascular disease has long been associated with high-fat diets and elevated levels of cholesterol—over 200 milligrams per deciliter of blood. When headache treatment consists of increased physical activity along with a diet rich in complex carbohydrates and low in fat, it has a significant preventive effect on the cardiovascular system. It can slow or stop the development of cardiovascular diseases such as hypertension, arteriosclerosis, and hypercholesterolemia, and it helps prevent heart attacks, strokes, and other serious conditions.

Fibromyalgia and Chronic Fatigue Syndrome

Constant excessive tiredness, muscle pain, and depression characterize these diseases. People with these ailments have low levels of serotonin, which may be the result of lifestyle factors.

Arthritis, Gout, and Other Inflammations of the Joints

These diseases can be treated successfully with lifestyle modification, because lifestyle has an effect on the body's production of chemicals that cause inflammation. These include histamines, substance P, and leukotrienes, all of which are elevated during headaches.

Osteoporosis

Osteoporosis, a condition that causes loss of bone mass, shares many common lifestyle factors with headaches. One of the most significant causes of osteoporosis is lack of physical activity. Other causes include smoking, excessive consumption of alcohol and caffeine, and lack of calcium retention, which is exacerbated by consuming large amounts of animal protein. All these factors closely mirror those identified as headache triggers.

Gallstones

Gallstones are lumps of cholesterol that form in the gall-bladder and cause severe discomfort or pain. One of the main reasons for their formation is a deficiency of fiber in the diet. Obesity and a high-calorie diet are other strong risk factors. Thus, the low-fat/high-complex-carbohydrate diet that I recommend for headache prevention will greatly reduce your risk of developing gallstones.

Cancer

A diet that is low in fat and high in complex carbohydrates naturally contains more vitamins, minerals, fibers, phytochemicals, and other components that help prevent cancer. Similarly, studies have shown a strong connection between physical activity and cancer and between stress and cancer. Thus, the lifestyle modifications that prevent headaches will also help fight this life-threatening disease.

Psychological Disorders

Low levels of serotonin can cause depression, anxiety, insomnia, and various other psychological disorders. In fact, antidepressants and similar medications artificially increase levels of serotonin in the blood. The lifestyle modifications recommended in this book will restore serotonin levels naturally without medication and thus reverse not only headaches, but also the related psychological disorders.

patients survived this procedure; but whether their headaches disappeared is unknown.

In Egypt and in Mesopotamia, which includes today's Iraq and is considered one of the cradles of civilization, people believed that headaches were caused by supernatural powers. Consequently, headaches were treated with prayers, chants, or spells. Even some of the gods seem to have suffered from headaches, including Zeus, the supreme god of Greek mythology, and the Egyptian god Horus.

Ancient Greece and Rome produced the first reliable and

systematic studies of headaches. Most distinguished physicians and scientists of that period of history studied and wrote about headaches. They include Hippocrates, who is called the father of modern medicine, and Galen, a second-century physician and writer whose work influenced much of European medicine until the nineteenth century. Galen introduced the term *hemikrania* (in Greek, *hemi* means half and *kranion* means skull) from which the word *migraine* was later derived. Aretaeus of Cappadocia, who lived in the second century AD, was the first to describe the symptoms of migraine.

Following the fall of the Roman Empire, Middle-Eastern scholars continued much of the scientific work. The most famous among them was Avicenna, an early-eleventh-century Persian physician, who provided new theories and insights to explain certain observations—for example, why particular smells, noises, or light sometimes triggered headaches. But medieval Europe was governed by strict Christian doctrines and was not ready to accept such thinking. Centuries would pass before scholars returned to the systematic study of headaches started by Galen.

Headache treatments have varied widely throughout the millennia. We know that prayers and chants have played a role since time immemorial. We also know that the ancient Greeks and Romans relied largely on herbal and other remedies derived from nature. In fact, this was true in many other cultures throughout the world. For example, Native Americans used to treat headaches with willow bark, which contains a substance similar to aspirin.

Some people believe there is a connection between headaches and a person's psychological state. More than 2,300 years ago, the Greek philosopher Plato noted that there seemed to be a correlation between the occurrence of headaches and certain emotions. Much later, the Austrian neurologist and founder of psychoanalysis Sigmund Freud contended that headaches were the result of some inner subconscious conflict.

Modern medicine has given us invaluable insights into the headache problem. It has uncovered a number of biochemical imbalances in the body that cause headaches, and it has produced various treatments, mostly in the form of medication, to correct some of these imbalances. It has also produced a number of advanced pain relievers. Yet, these solutions are far from satisfactory. There is no "silver bullet," no magic pill or conventional treatment that will reliably prevent or eliminate headaches.

THE HEADACHE PROBLEM TODAY

Although headaches are not life threatening, they are extremely costly emotionally and financially. Even an occasional mild headache is disturbing enough to make work more difficult or to take the enjoyment out of your favorite leisure activity. A severe headache can be completely debilitating, preventing the sufferer from doing any work or routine activity. In addition, depression and irritability frequently accompany chronic headaches, which may impose a burden on the patient's family and lead to a significantly decreased quality of life.

Chronic headache disorders cause much greater impairment of function than had previously been suspected. The reality is that patients with chronic headaches may be able to function physically, but they function at a level considerably below their capabilities. The level of impairment in terms of lost productivity or the ability to take care of everyday needs is similar to that of patients with cardiovascular diseases. Many studies have been conducted to assess the overall impact of headaches on society, including medical costs, lost work time, family relationships, and quality of life. Although results vary widely due to different methods of gathering data and evaluation, even the most conservative estimates confirm that headaches present an enormous problem whose burden cannot be underestimated. Here are some staggering statistics:

- According to a 1989 survey of a sample population in the United States, 95 percent of women and 91 percent of men suffer from headaches at some point during their lifetime.

- A survey conducted in Denmark in 1987 determined that 19 percent of adults had suffered from at least one headache during the fourteen-day period before the survey. A survey in the United Kingdom revealed similar results in 1971.

- Nearly 10 million people in the United States suffer from regular migraine headaches; and 40 percent of people in North America have occasional migraines.

- A study in Nigeria concluded that 60 percent of university students have recurrent headaches.

- On average, 55 percent of migraine sufferers miss two workdays per month. In addition, 88 percent of sufferers work more than five days per month despite having a migraine.

- Approximately 85 percent of female migraine sufferers and 77 percent of male migraine sufferers see a physician at some point for their migraine headaches.

- It is estimated that 5 to 10 percent of North Americans occasionally seek medical help for relief from disabling headaches.

- In the United States, headaches cost an estimated $50 billion each year. The cost to business in lost productivity is approximately $6 billion to $17 billion a year.

HEADACHE TREATMENTS

There are many headache treatments, including over-the-counter medications, prescription drugs, and a variety of alternative treatments. For secondary headaches, conventional medical treatments focus on eliminating the underlying organic disorder or disease that is causing the headaches. Primary headaches do not have any such disorders associated with them, and so they are usually treated with pain relievers. Unfortunately, this does not prevent them from recurring. Most books on this subject state that headaches, especially migraines, are a chronic condition that cannot be prevented or cured; they can only be managed by a variety of approaches, the most common of which is the use of medication. The following sections discuss some of these approaches and why they are not always effective in eliminating chronic headaches.

Over-the-Counter Medications

If you suffer from headaches and have consulted a physician about the problem, chances are you have not found a satisfactory solution. In fact, most headache sufferers do not seek professional medical help on a regular basis. They may think their headaches are not serious enough to warrant a visit to the doctor, they may feel there is no solution for their problem, or they may not be able to afford medical treatment. Whatever the reason, the fact is that the majority of headache sufferers treat themselves with over-the-counter medications.

Many of these drugs provide temporary relief from headache pain. Nevertheless, despite the large number of product names, there are only three essential ingredients in all nonprescription pain relievers—*aspirin, acetaminophen,* and *ibuprofen.* The only differences are in their quantity and combination, and sometimes in the addition of caffeine, which can improve the effectiveness of the medication. To give you some examples: Anacin, Bufferin, Midol, and, of course, Bayer Aspirin all contain the chemical aspirin; Anacin-3, Excedrin PM, Panadol, and Tylenol contain the chemical acetaminophen; Advil, Medipren, Motrin, and Nuprin contain the chemical ibuprofen; and Extra Strength Excedrin and Excedrin Migraine are a combination of aspirin, acetaminophen, and caffeine. Product labels will list exactly what you are taking, but you should be aware of the possible problems associated with each chemical.

The most common and potentially serious problem associated with the use of aspirin and ibuprofen is irritation of the stomach and the intestines. Initially, the irritation may seem to be a simple stomach upset, but it can lead to internal bleeding and other problems. Acetaminophen does not cause this problem, and therefore it is one of the few pain relievers that can be given to children. But the overuse of these so-called simple medications can lead to long-term complications such as liver or kidney damage, increased blood pressure, nausea, ringing in the ears, and a host of other medical complications.

One of the most difficult problems associated with even the simplest pain relievers is the *rebound headache.* How do rebound headaches develop? When people take large doses of a medication regularly and frequently, the body develops a dependence on and a tolerance to the medication. As the pain-free periods between headaches become shorter and shorter, the medication must be taken more and more frequently and in increasing amounts. The result is a cycle of ever-increasing pain and medication. In the end, the medication that was supposed to relieve the pain has become one of its main causes.

Prescription Medications

If your headaches are severe and frequent, simple pain relievers may not provide much relief. Many prescription medications relieve headaches, but only an experienced physician or pharmacist can provide adequate advice on their use. There are two important points to consider if you take prescription medications. First, all headache medications can cause side effects. Depending on the type and combination of medications, side effects range from problems such as nausea, dizziness, or diarrhea to potentially life-threatening conditions. In addition, many drugs lose their effectiveness over time. Some drugs are addictive, and, as in the case of simple pain relievers, they can lead to rebound headaches.

Regular use of headache medications also tends to lower the headache threshold, or the level of tolerance beyond which a headache occurs. This increased sensitivity to possible headache triggers brings on more headaches and the need for additional medication.

The second point about prescription medications concerns some specific anti-migraine drugs, many of which have come on the market in the last few years. All these drugs share a common link with *serotonin,* a chemical in our bloodstream that plays an important role in preventing headaches. The drugs either directly mimic the actions of serotonin or cause similar effects, notably constricting blood vessels and reducing inflammation. This is true of the most widely prescribed drugs such as *sumatriptan* (found in Imitrex and Imigran), *dihydroergotamine* (DHE 45), or *ergotamine tartrate* (Cafergot, Wigraine, Ergostat). Regulating levels of serotonin is undoubtedly important in controlling headaches. But instead of using specialized drugs with their limitations and side effects, you can control serotonin levels by natural means, such as lifestyle modification.

Alternative Treatments

There are many unconventional and supplemental treatments for headaches. Some date back centuries, and others were developed as a result of recent experiments. The treatments are too numerous to list, but we can group them into several major categories. These include relaxation and exercise-based treatments, nutritional and herbal approaches, and a variety of miscellaneous therapies.

Relaxation and exercise are essential to a healthy life and may alleviate a number of headaches, especially milder forms of tension headaches. They are also fundamental components of the lifestyle modification treatment, which is aimed at preventing more severe headaches.

Nutritional approaches to headache treatment generally focus on the elimination of specific foods or the addition of certain nutrients, vitamins, or minerals. The first group includes various elimination diets, which call for the exclusion of specific foods that may trigger headaches. But although there are some known headache triggers in food, elimination diets are not very effective treatments because most headaches are caused by a number of factors and cannot be alleviated by the absence of a few substances.

Supplemental approaches to treating headaches typically focus on increasing the intake of certain vitamins and minerals. Of course, appropriate levels of vitamins and minerals are necessary for good health whether or not you suffer from headaches. And although a well-balanced diet provides most essential vitamins and minerals, dietary supplements are often beneficial, especially during the period of transition to a healthier lifestyle.

Herbal approaches to headache treatment have existed for centuries. Several herbs, for example, bay (*Laurus nobilis*), feverfew (*Tanacetum parthenium*), and willow bark (*Salicis cortex*), are remedies whose effectiveness has been verified through controlled scientific studies. Many herbs used for headache treatment work like mild pain relievers. Other herbs attempt to correct some of the biochemical imbalances that may cause headaches. Of course, herbal remedies cannot eliminate or prevent the lifestyle-related factors that create headaches. However, many herbs have a beneficial effect on general health, and they can be used in combination with the various lifestyle modifications described in this book.

In summary, most unconventional approaches have not been tested in controlled clinical trials, which makes it difficult to evaluate them objectively. Undoubtedly, some approaches work and others do not. If you find relief in any of these methods and they are not harmful to your health, continue using them. But the fact that you are reading this book suggests that you have not yet found a satisfactory solution for your headache problem.

The Lifestyle Modification Approach

As already stated, headaches are very complex problems. And because they are strongly connected to a person's lifestyle, no single action or treatment is likely to provide a lasting solution. To illustrate this by analogy, consider your garden. If it becomes infested with harmful insects, you may reach for a pesticide as a quick fix. This eliminates unwanted pests, but it also eliminates ladybugs and other useful insects that keep aphids and other parasites in check. Without these insects, you may have an even bigger problem, requiring more insecticide and starting a cycle of an ecological imbalance. What was missing from your garden in the first place? Lizards and birds that would have controlled the insect population. But you cannot introduce such animals by simply releasing them in the garden. Instead, you must create the right environment in which they can emerge and thrive naturally.

Your body is an ecosystem. It needs a great number of minerals, vitamins, hormones, and other biochemical components to keep its organs and subsystems working properly. Despite all the medical research to date, we still do not completely understand some of the biochemical processes that keep the body functioning. Nonetheless, it is clear that the body has a strong need to keep all its components and functions in balance. Its tendency to maintain internal stability is called *homeostasis*. A headache is a sign that the body is experiencing an imbalance that it cannot repair on its own. Treating your headache with a medication that alters the level of a particular chemical in the body is similar to using pesticides in your garden. Obviously, we must learn a new approach to headache treatment—an approach that treats the body's complete ecosystem.

Lifestyle modification focuses on gradually restoring

your body's ecosystem to a natural healthy state. This requires balanced nutrition, adequate physical activity, and relief from stress. However, lifestyle modification is not based on prescribing a specific diet, exercise regimen, or other structured program. Rather, it teaches you how to adopt and enjoy a healthy lifestyle.

The lifestyle modification approach has its roots in a clinical study that I conducted at Loma Linda University's School of Public Health. The Loma Linda study, which is discussed in Chapter 2, demonstrated that there is a very strong connection between high-fat diets and migraine headaches. This was the first step toward a radically new way of dealing with headaches—that is, focusing on headache prevention by eliminating the lifestyle-related causes of headaches. These insights inspired the development of a comprehensive set of techniques and strategies to teach headache patients how to change old habits and adhere to a new, healthier lifestyle.

Given the existing headache classifications, you may feel that in order to find the right treatment, it is essential to identify the type of headaches you suffer from. This is the case with secondary headaches, whose real cause is rooted in some other disease or disorder. If you suspect that this might be the case, you should consult your physician to obtain proper diagnosis and treatment. The vast majority of headaches, however, are of the primary nature—migraines, tension headaches, and cluster headaches. Since these headaches are not caused by organic problems, the treatment options offered by conventional medicine are limited. The lifestyle modification approach is an attractive alternative, and it has proven highly effective in treating migraines and most other common headaches. Thus, to benefit from this program, it is not essential to determine whether your headache is a migraine or one of the other primary headaches. Remember that many patients suffer from multiple forms of headaches.

One of my first patients provides a good example of

what could be termed a "difficult-headache patient." His headaches had most of the symptoms of a migraine, sometimes with an aura, but the pain was usually centered right behind one of his eyes—a classic symptom of a cluster headache. Occasionally, his headaches seemed to be tension headaches. Given the multitude of different symptoms, he consulted his primary physician, who found no organic disorder. His doctor gave him some very general advice—eliminate certain types of foods, take relaxing walks and showers, and reduce stress. But without specific guidelines or strategies to bring about any significant changes in his lifestyle, the advice was of little help.

This patient was a perfect candidate for my lifestyle modification approach, which greatly diminished the severity and frequency of his headaches. In fact, unless your headaches are the result of an injury, tumor, or some other organic disorder, a lifestyle modification approach is very likely to alleviate your headaches and improve your general health and quality of life.

CONCLUSION

As you see, there are many headache treatments, and most rely on medication. Although headache medications can help temporarily, in the long run they cannot prevent headaches from recurring. But there are steps you can take that will eliminate your headache problems. Before we study the details of my lifestyle modification plan, we will examine what happens to the body before and during a headache, and we will discuss why lifestyle has such an impact on our health and well-being.

CHAPTER 2

My Search for the Ideal Treatment

Making the simple complicated is commonplace;
making the complicated simple, awesomely simple—
that's creativity.

—Charles Mingus

O ne of the most frustrating things about headaches is the multitude of seemingly unrelated factors that can cause them. A recent scientific study that I conducted at Loma Linda University is the basis for a completely new approach to headache treatment. The study offered insights into the complex biochemistry of migraine headaches, which enabled me to tie together the various known causes of migraines and demonstrate that the seemingly unrelated factors that cause headaches are in fact related. This led to the development of a radically new approach to headache treatment, based on gradual lifestyle modification, that is highly effective in preventing not only migraines, but also most other common forms of headache. This chapter describes my search for this new headache treatment and explains the fundamental connection between lifestyle, body chemistry, and headaches.

THE INITIAL IDEA

All scientific research requires time, effort, resources, talent, dedication, and, last but not least, luck. Many important medical discoveries, including x-rays, anesthetics, insulin, and penicillin, were the result of serendipity. Similarly, a drug or treatment developed and used for a certain illness may have a surprisingly beneficial impact on an entirely different and unrelated condition. One of the best examples of this is common aspirin. This synthetic chemical has been used to treat pain for over 100 years; but it was only recently that physicians discovered the effectiveness of aspirin in preventing heart attacks, strokes, and other coronary problems.

The headache treatment described in this book also has its roots in accidental discovery. The initial idea began to develop at a medical practice specializing in preventive care and lifestyle medicine, where patients with type II diabetes were put on a low-fat diet. When they returned for a follow-up visit, we found that their diabetic symptoms had improved. In addition, some patients who had suffered from migraine headaches before beginning the diet noted that their headaches had become less frequent and less severe.

This unexpected side effect of the low-fat diet roused my interest. During the 1980s, I had worked as a physician in the area of neurology. Part of my work included the treatment of migraine headaches from a purely neurological point of view. But I had always harbored a belief that most chronic diseases could be prevented, or their symptoms minimized, through appropriate lifestyle modification. I believed that most headaches were manifestations of a lifestyle-related imbalance, and the results of the diabetes treatment convinced me that I was right. This gave me the incentive to do further research in hope of supporting my conviction.

The First Headache Patient

After the amazing experience with the diabetes patients, I

recommended a low-fat/high-complex-carbohydrate diet to one of my migraine patients. I also helped him develop some basic strategies to maintain a fat intake of 20 to 30 grams per day—approximately 10 to 15 percent of his total caloric intake—and to increase his intake of complex carbohydrates. After three weeks on this new dietary regimen, the patient did indeed observe a dramatic decrease in the occurrence and severity of his headaches. This was enough to garner great excitement and warrant further, more systematic research.

Medical Literature Search

Any serious scientific experiment must start with a thorough examination of prior research related to the subject. When I began to search for scientific articles that established a connection between migraine headaches and a low-fat diet, I was surprised to find that no such studies had been published. Although a number of studies revealed a possible connection between diet and migraine headaches, most focused on specific chemicals that seemed to play a role in the occurrence of migraines, such as *tyramine* or *aspartame*. Eliminating specific food products containing these chemicals—for example, red wine and aged cheese—from the patient's diet was the recommended treatment for migraines. Unfortunately, elimination diets have never proven very effective in practice, and most patients who experiment with this approach become very discouraged. In fact, many of the participants in the Loma Linda University study asked if the prescribed treatment would be an elimination diet. They had been through this depressing experience and were unhappy with the results. Not only had their diets been highly restricted, they continued to suffer from headaches. The failure of elimination diets indicates that focusing on specific chemicals in the diet does not provide a satisfactory solution to the headache problem.

During my investigation of diet and headaches, I found

many studies suggesting that the fatty substances contained in our blood might cause migraines. Indeed, levels of free fatty acids in the blood are considerably elevated during migraine attacks. This provided an important clue in my quest to find a better headache treatment. But more questions arose from this discovery than were answered. Does the increased blood fat cause the headaches or is it the other way around? If blood fat is the cause of headaches, why does it become elevated and how can it be lowered? What about those headaches that do not seem to have any connection with fat triggers, such as those caused by stress or the consumption of red wine? After much more research, I was able to answer some of these questions, and a clear picture of the headache problem began to emerge. It was becoming increasingly evident that most headaches are triggered by the same biochemical imbalances in the body, but these imbalances can be caused by many different factors.

HOW LIFESTYLE HABITS CAUSE HEADACHES

There are hundreds of studies in scientific literature linking headaches to external factors as well as to different biochemical imbalances in the body. As part of my research at Loma Linda University, I created a diagram that I call the *Theoretical Model of a Headache.* The diagram, shown in Figure 2.1 on page 29, brings together the findings of many different scientific studies and illustrates the underlying biochemical processes that can cause headaches. The headache model will serve as the basis for the lifestyle modification approach presented in this book.

Habits That Affect Blood Chemistry

A headache is generally preceded by a narrowing of the blood vessels that surround the brain, or *vasoconstriction.* This is followed by the dilation of the blood vessels, or *vasodilatation,* which is believed to cause the head pain.

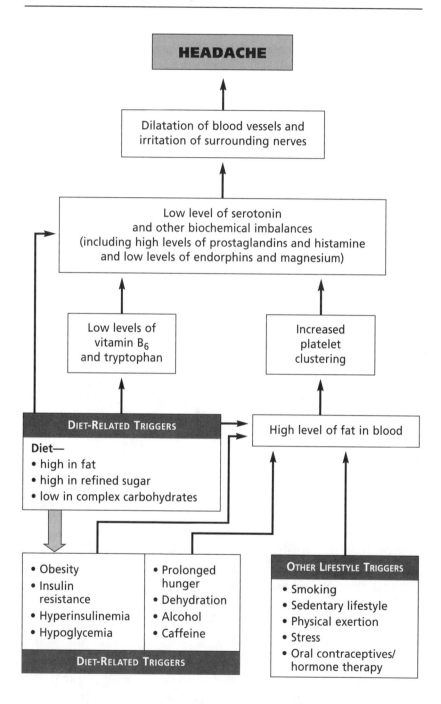

Figure 2.1. Theoretical Model of a Headache

There are two possible explanations for this. One theory suggests that the dilated blood vessels press on sensitive nerve ends. The other theorizes that headache pain is caused by inflammation of the area around the blood vessels. Regardless of which explanation is true, vasodilatation and headache usually occur together and are preceded by specific biochemical imbalances in the body.

One of the main culprits is an abnormally low level of serotonin in the body. Other important substances that influence blood vessels and blood flow in the brain include prostaglandins, histamine, endorphins, magnesium, and many others. Serotonin is a messenger—a *neurotransmitter* in medical terminology—that carries information from nerve ends to different parts in the body, where it is detected by special receptors and causes a wide range of reactions. Among other things, serotonin is involved in controlling depression, anxiety, and eating and sleeping patterns. But serotonin also prevents blood vessels from dilating too much. Therefore, when levels of serotonin are low, the blood vessels dilate, which generally brings on a headache. In fact, another term for migraine headache is *low-serotonin syndrome.* Let us now examine the factors that cause serotonin levels to fall.

Two important conditions determine low serotonin levels. One is a lack of vitamin B_6 and *tryptophan,* and the other is a high degree of platelet clustering. Tryptophan is an essential building block in the production of serotonin, which, in turn, requires the presence of vitamin B_6. Low levels of tryptophan result in low levels of serotonin. Vitamin B_6 and tryptophan are present in many fruits, vegetables, grains, and legumes.

To understand the second reason for low levels of serotonin—*platelet clustering*—it will be helpful to understand the basic makeup of blood. Blood consists of a clear liquid called *plasma,* which contains a variety of different particles. Most people are familiar with two of these particles—*red blood cells,* which give blood its red color and are responsible for transporting oxygen and nutrients throughout the body; and *white blood cells,* which enable the body to fight against infection. The particles we are most interested in are called *platelets.* These tiny round or oval-shaped discs— about one ten-thousandth of an inch in diameter—function as biochemical storehouses for enzymes and other substances, including serotonin.

Platelets usually travel freely and smoothly through the blood vessels. But under certain conditions, platelets start to *aggregate,* or cluster. When this happens, the platelet walls become damaged, and the chemicals stored there, such as serotonin, start to leak into the blood. The additional serotonin temporarily increases constriction of the blood vessels, and it is during this period that some people sense a headache coming on or experience an aura. But shortly thereafter, the serotonin is degraded and eliminated from the body. And without sufficient serotonin to constrict the blood vessels, vasodilatation and an accompanying headache are the results.

The main cause of increased platelet clustering is a growth in levels of certain fatty substances in the bloodstream. The two main groups are *blood lipids,* which include cholesterol and triglycerides, and several different types of *free fatty acids,* including *stearic, linoleic, palmitic,* and *oleic acids.* Free fatty acids and blood lipids are mutually connected, and the levels of one generally influence the levels of the others. To simplify our discussion, we will use the phrase *blood fat* to refer to both groups.

The reason for increased platelet clustering in the presence of fat is easy to understand. Added fat changes the consistency and flow properties of blood so that it becomes thicker. Picture the difference between water and oil. Both are liquids, but water flows more easily than oil. The blood-thickening effect occurs because fat in the blood takes up space in the blood vessels and leaves less room for other particles to maneuver. This makes it easier for the platelets to cluster.

When I realized that high levels of blood fat were one of the main causes of headaches, I began to investigate possible environmental and lifestyle factors that may increase levels of blood fat. It turned out that almost all known headache triggers cause blood-fat levels to rise. Therefore, blood fat is the common denominator of all conditions known to cause headaches.

High-Fat, High-Sugar, Low-Complex-Carbohydrate Diets

The food we eat directly and immediately affects fat levels and other nutrients in the bloodstream. A high-fat diet will cause a rise in levels of blood fat, and any sugar we consume is transferred into the bloodstream. In order to understand the impact of blood sugar on levels of blood fat, we must first know how the body processes and uses sugar.

We eat many types of sugar, all of which are broken down by digestive processes into one of the simplest forms of sugar, called *glucose,* or blood sugar. A rise in blood sugar triggers the release of *insulin,* a natural hormone that helps metabolize sugar into energy and influences the metabolism of fat in the body. Thus, insulin reduces blood sugar to normal levels. This is what occurs when we eat natural sugars such as those contained in fruits, vegetables, or other unprocessed foods.

Unfortunately, the most common form of sugar consumed today is pure *sucrose,* which is a combination of two simple sugars, glucose and *fructose.* Sucrose does occur naturally in many fruits and plants, but it never occurs by itself. It must be extracted from plants, usually from sugarcane or sugar beets, which have the highest concentrations of sucrose. This involves crushing the sugarcane or sugar beets and repeatedly boiling and cooling the juice while adding various chemicals to crystallize the sucrose. The process removes all proteins, minerals, vitamins, and other natural substances. What remains is pure white sugar.

Since sucrose does not occur in this highly concentrated form in nature, the body has difficulty processing it. When you ingest a large amount, it quickly enters the bloodstream and causes the release of an unnaturally high amount of insulin to deal with the excess blood sugar, or *hyperglycemia.* This removes the additional sugar, but since there is too much insulin, the reaction continues for too long a period. The result is a state of low blood sugar, which causes levels of blood fat to rise. Now we can see the link between blood sugar and blood fat. In short, whenever the level of blood sugar is insufficient to serve as the body's fuel, more fat is released into the bloodstream to fill the gap.

Low blood sugar also causes the release of several hormones, notably *adrenaline.* This increases platelet clustering and changes the body's metabolism, which intensifies the effect of the increased blood fat and brings on a headache. It is interesting to note that at one time migraines were called *hypoglycemic headaches,* or low blood-sugar headaches.

Another important substance that links a high-fat diet with headaches is a group of fatty substances called *prostaglandins,* which are produced by most body tissues. Like cholesterol, there are "good" and "bad" types of prostaglandins. The latter, called Series-1 prostaglandins, or simply PGE-1, are potent vasodilators.

Levels of prostaglandins can be influenced in two ways. First, a proper ratio of omega-3 oils—found, for example, in fish, flaxseeds, or walnuts—to omega-6 oils—found, for example, in margarine—can keep prostaglandins in balance. Of course, nutrition is an essential factor in influencing the balance of these fats in the body. The second factor influencing levels of prostaglandins is serotonin. The release of serotonin into the bloodstream causes prostaglandin levels to rise. This naturally doubles the risk for headache because both serotonin and prostaglandins are strong vasodilators.

Diet-Related Chronic Disorders

A diet high in fat and refined sugar and low in complex carbohydrates is one of the main factors in the development of several chronic disorders that are also linked to headaches. *Obesity* is one of the most common of these conditions. It is characterized by an excessive amount of fat stored in the body as well as an excessive amount of fat circulating in the bloodstream. The chronically increased levels of blood fat explain why obesity is considered a precondition for headaches.

Another common disorder related to nutrition is *insulin resistance.* As the name suggests, it describes a condition in which insulin can no longer process blood sugar. Thus, despite the fact that the body may produce adequate or even excessive amounts of insulin—a disorder called *hyper-insulinemia*—blood-sugar levels remain high. But because the body is unable to use the sugar as fuel, it increases its levels of blood fat to provide additional or alternate fuel. This leads to increased platelet clustering, a reduction of serotonin, and headache.

Chronic *hypoglycemia,* or low blood sugar, is another disorder frequently linked to headaches because insufficient levels of blood sugar force the body to use more fat as fuel. Thus, chronic hypoglycemia has the same harmful effect as the insulin-related disorders described above.

Other Diet-Related Headache Triggers

Although a diet rich in fat and refined sugar and low in complex carbohydrates is a major cause of headaches, there are four other diet-related headache triggers—prolonged hunger, dehydration, alcohol, and caffeine. All four bring about a rise in blood-fat levels.

Prolonged hunger is similar to chronic hypoglycemia in that it produces a temporary state of low blood sugar, and since no new sugars are supplied as food, the body must use its stored fat for fuel. The corresponding rise in blood fat then follows the now familiar path toward headache.

Another potent headache trigger is dehydration. The reason is quite simple. Lack of water increases the viscosity of the blood so that it becomes thicker. Therefore, it does not flow as easily, and this increases the likelihood that platelets will stick together and become damaged. Unlike some other triggers, dehydration does not increase the total amount of blood fat, but it does increase its concentration. Lack of fluid is especially critical after meals because many nutrients require water to transport and metabolize food and to store it in the form of fat. When you do not drink water with your meal, your body must use the fluid currently available in the bloodstream. This further increases fat concentration, reduces the blood's flow properties, and increases platelet clustering.

Alcohol is one of the most potent and reliable headache triggers. First, alcohol is a vasodilator—and remember that vasodilatation is a common precondition of headache. Second, alcohol interferes with the function of the liver, which regulates the metabolism of carbohydrates. As a result, it has a hypoglycemic effect on the body, which results in an increase of blood fat. Finally, when alcohol is metabolized and removed from the body, the byproduct of the chemical reaction is fat, which is then added to the bloodstream.

Caffeine, which is found naturally in coffee, some teas, and many soft drinks, is a potent vasoconstrictor. When used infrequently and in small amounts, it can actually be used as a headache medication. A cup of coffee taken at the onset of a headache can sometimes abort it. Caffeine is also added to some pain relievers to improve their effectiveness. But in larger quantities and when consumed habitually— generally more than three cups of coffee per day—caffeine significantly increases levels of blood fat, notably cholesterol. It also increases platelet clustering. As we know, high blood fat and platelet clustering contribute to the degradation of serotonin, which leads to vasodilatation and headache.

Caffeine can also cause headaches via another mechanism—the withdrawal effect. When you use caffeine regularly over extended periods, your body adapts to its presence in the bloodstream by compensating for its constricting effect. The sudden interruption of a regular caffeine supply does not give the body enough time to discontinue the compensation, which results in excessive vasodilatation and the development of a headache.

Other Lifestyle-Related Triggers

There is a connection between headaches and many other factors that increase levels of blood fat. The ills of smoking are well documented. Among the many problems and risks, smoking is known to cause headaches or to exacerbate their symptoms. Smoking increases levels of LDL—the "bad" cholesterol—but it also increases the blood's viscosity and platelet clustering, which can encourage the formation of blood clots.

Another critical factor in controlling headaches is physical activity. It is important to realize that a lack of physical activity, as well as too much of it, may bring about a rise in levels of blood fat. A sedentary lifestyle has a profound effect on the body's metabolism, making it difficult to clear fat from the bloodstream. At the other extreme, excessive exercise induces a temporary state of hypoglycemia because it depletes the body's sugar reserves. The depletion of blood sugar forces the body to increase the level of fat in the blood in order to provide the necessary fuel to muscles and other tissues.

Stress is another well-known headache trigger. Chronic stress can cause a number of biochemical imbalances, which the body tries to correct. Psychological or emotional problems—for example, those resulting from overwhelming amounts of work, difficult relationships, or financial worries—are common sources of stress. A multitude of environmental or physical pressures—including injury, pollution, lack of oxygen, hypothermia, and hyperthermia—can also cause a stress response.

Like all the other triggers discussed so far, stress causes blood-fat levels to rise. In the case of physical or environmental triggers, the body provides additional fuel to cope with the stress situation. In the case of psychological stress triggers, the body prepares itself for a fight-or-flight response to a perceived danger by providing the necessary fuel for the expected physical activity. Unfortunately, stress in our civilized society is rarely relieved by a physical fight or by running away, and so the increased fat remains in the bloodstream. You may already be aware that stress causes a rise in cholesterol, which is one type of fat. In fact, prolonged stress causes an accumulation of all types of fats in the blood.

Finally, some oral contraceptives and some types of hormonal therapy may produce headaches. This applies particularly to products containing high levels of estrogen. By now you may have guessed the reason. Yes, once again, fat is the culprit. Fluctuations in estrogen levels influence the amount of fat in the blood and cause headaches.

THE BIG PICTURE

As you can see in Figure 2.1 on page 29, several paths lead to the occurrence of headaches. Each path is the result of a number of biochemical imbalances in the body. The goal of headache prevention is to disrupt these pathways by correcting some of the imbalances. Conventional medical science tries to target one or more of the specific imbalances with drug intervention. In fact, if you look at the following list of conventional headache treatments, you will find that each one corresponds directly with one of the boxes in Figure 2.1:

- Drugs that constrict blood vessels attempt to counteract vasodilatation.

- Serotonin injections boost the body's serotonin levels to prevent vasodilatation.

- Vitamin B_6 and tryptophan improve the production of serotonin.

- Drugs that decrease platelet clustering, such as aspirin, prevent platelet damage and the resulting elimination of serotonin from the body.

- Drugs that reduce levels of blood fat reduce platelet clustering.

Several other drugs or interventions used for headache treatment attempt to correct other known headache-related imbalances, such as deficiencies of magnesium and certain vitamins. But the main problem with any intervention that tries to correct the imbalance of one chemical substance in the body is that it is impossible to do this in isolation. Why? Most substances fluctuate with other substances and biochemical processes as part of a complex chain of interactions. Imagine a complex network of springs, ropes, and pulleys of various lengths and strengths. Changing any of these components will affect the immediate neighborhood, and send shock waves through the entire network until it again reaches a stable state. The human body is an extremely complex network of biochemical reactions. Due to the many dependencies and mutual interactions, changing the level of one substance generally affects the levels of many others.

Can we possibly hope for an intervention that will restore all the body's natural biochemical balances to prevent headaches? The answer is yes. But this will not happen by focusing on specific imbalances. Instead, we must rely on the body's own self-regulating abilities. Each simple stimulus, such as hunger, fright, or just getting up from a chair, sets in motion a chain reaction of complex biochemical processes that regulate heart rate, blood pressure, oxygen and nutrient supplies, and great many other things. Figure 2.1 establishes a link between headaches and external stimuli, or lifestyle factors. Thus, it provides the basis for a new treatment—a gradual lifestyle modification that eliminates harmful stimuli and allows the body to restore and maintain its internal biochemical balances.

THE LOMA LINDA UNIVERSITY STUDY

I conducted a study of headaches at Loma Linda University's School of Public Health in California from 1994 to 1996. The main purpose of the study was to determine whether a low-fat, high-complex-carbohydrate diet could lower the frequency, intensity, and duration of migraine headaches. It was intended as the first step toward a new, systematic approach to headache treatment using lifestyle modification. The findings of the study were first published in two scientific journals—*Medical Hypothesis* and the *Journal of Women's Health and Gender-Based Medicine*—but since the improvements were so dramatic, a number of popular magazines also featured articles about this new treatment.

Organization of the Study

The study was conducted over a twelve-week period and was divided into three 4-week segments. The first was called the *baseline period*. During this time, patients were asked not to change anything in their eating or other habits, but to keep detailed food and headache diaries. Our purpose was to collect data that we would be able to compare to data gathered at the end of the study.

The first intervention occurred at the end of the baseline period. This was a consultation with each patient that lasted one hour and focused on his or her diary. Based on a computer-aided nutritional evaluation, we gave patients reading materials and specific strategies for changing their eating habits. Our objective was to reduce their fat consumption to 20 to 30 grams per day, or approximately 10 to 15 percent of their total calories. The various step-by-step strategies, to be discussed later in this book, focused on how to combat hunger, how to estimate the amount of fat consumed, and how to change the basic composition of meals to reach the goal. At the end of the baseline period, we took measurements of each patient's body fat and weight, and conducted blood tests. We asked patients to continue keeping their headache and food diaries for the remainder of the experiment.

The next individual consultation, lasting thirty minutes, took place after the next four-week period, the *transition period*. The main purpose of this consultation was to determine how successfully the patients had made the transition to the new eating patterns and to gauge if they were able to maintain the lifestyle change. Patients were given suggestions tailored individually to their specific problems to help them make the transition as effortless and unobtrusive as possible.

The last meeting took place at the end of the third four-week period, the *final phase*. During this meeting, we again measured patients' body fat and weight, and repeated the blood tests for comparison purposes.

Results of the Study

The outcome of the experiment surpassed even the most optimistic expectations. It demonstrated a very strong connection between high fat intake and migraine headaches. Patients who had decreased their fat intake had significantly lowered the frequency, intensity, and duration of their migraine headaches. Consequently, they were able to minimize or discontinue their intake of pain medication.

Headache *frequency* refers to the number of headaches per month. The participants in the study had, on average, almost nine migraine headaches during the baseline period. However, at the end of the study, headache frequency had been reduced to an average of just over two times per month. This represents an astonishing improvement of nearly 71 percent.

We measured headache *intensity* using a rating scale. Patients were asked to give each headache a number from zero to five, where zero meant no headache and five corresponded to an extremely intense, incapacitating headache. Before the low-fat/high-complex-carbohydrate intervention, patients reported an average headache intensity close to three. But by the end of the study, this dropped to below one. That is, headache intensity decreased by about 66 percent.

Headache *duration* is nearly impossible to measure directly since headaches sometimes originate or end in the middle of sleep, and the exact starting or ending times are unknown. For that reason, a special measure, called the *headache index*, was invented, which reliably reflects headache duration. The diet intervention resulted in a 74-percent decrease in the average duration of pain.

Medication intake was determined by the number of days per month that patients took headache medication. Before starting the low-fat/high-complex-carbohydrate diet, patients took pain medication of various kinds approximately ten times per month. At the end study, pain medication use dropped to only three times a month—a decrease of 72 percent.

The above numbers are, of course, only averages; and you may be wondering if you too will be able to find relief using the treatment described in this book. The following additional statistics should help:

- Nearly all participants, 94 percent, reported at least a 40-percent improvement in the frequency, intensity, and duration of their headaches. Almost half the participants, 48 percent, reported at least a 90-percent improvement, and many were headache-free.

- Only a small fraction of participants, 6 percent, reported little or no noticeable improvement in their condition.

We made several other interesting observations. Before the study, patients had consumed an average of 67 grams of fat per day, with some eating as many as 120 grams per day. This is not very difficult to do. For example, a single slice of cheesecake or a double cheeseburger can contain as many as 60 grams of fat. During the eight-week study period, patients reduced their fat intake to around 27 grams of fat per day. This was approximately a 60-percent decrease in fat intake.

As a direct consequence of this reduction, other positive changes occurred as well. In particular, patients' total caloric intake decreased by an average of 32 percent, and their cholesterol levels decreased from an average of 206 to 178. Other nutritional components such as minerals and vitamins increased because patients were eating more fruit, vegetables, grains, legumes, and fiber. Furthermore, they had decreased their sodium intake. One side effect of the headache treatment, which most participants welcomed, was a slight weight loss. On average, patients decreased their body fat by 4 percent. Finally, most patients reported having a feeling of well-being and a better quality of life.

The results of the Loma Linda University study clearly show that balanced nutrition plays a major role in the prevention of headaches. This finding contradicts studies claiming that nutrition has little or no impact on headaches. However, these studies considered different types of food groups and their influence on headaches. That is, the food groups had been chosen not by the amount of total fat, but by the levels of other substances, such as tyramine. Since all food groups had similar amounts of fat, it is not surprising that researchers found no significant connection with headaches.

CONCLUSION

The Loma Linda University study demonstrated beyond a doubt that a low-fat/high-complex-carbohydrate diet significantly decreases the occurrence of headaches and, consequently, the use of pain medication. One of the most important contributions of the study was the identification of elevated amounts of blood fat as the common denominator of primary headaches. These findings established a connection between a multitude of seemingly unrelated headache triggers, all of which cause levels of blood fat to rise. This opened the way to a radically new treatment of headaches based on specific lifestyle modifications to reduce blood-fat levels and to restore the natural biochemical balances of the body.

CHAPTER 3

Nutrition and Headache

Thy food shall be thy medicine.

—Hippocrates

This chapter is about a subject that is very important to most people—food. As you have seen by the Loma Linda University study, there is an undeniable connection between nutrition and the recurrence of headaches. This is why a healthy diet is an essential part of my headache-prevention program. However, we will not ask you to give up things that you like to eat. Instead, your goal is to learn to enjoy healthful foods, which your body really needs, just as much you now enjoy a fat cheeseburger or a big piece of chocolate cake. "Impossible!" you think.

We acquire taste over time by exposure to different types of food. And although we generally develop our taste for certain types of food early in our childhood, we can learn to change it at any point later in life. Before presenting the strategies that will enable you to bring about changes in your preferences for certain foods, let us look at the long-term nutritional goals of my headache-prevention program.

NUTRITION AND BODY CHEMISTRY

The human body needs nutrients and other substances in order to live. These include fats, proteins, carbohydrates, vitamins, minerals, and water. Fats, protein, carbohydrates, and some minerals, including water, are considered *macro-nutrients* because the body requires them in large quantities for energy, growth, and maintenance. The body also needs small quantities of vitamins and minerals, or *micronutrients,* which it uses for growth, protection against disease, and good health.

The body produces some of these substances by itself, but it gets most of them in the form of food. This means we can influence the composition of our body and the way it functions by the types and amounts of food we eat. A healthy, well-balanced diet will automatically increase your intake of beneficial nutrients and decrease your intake of unwholesome foods that may cause headaches and other problems. What is a healthy diet? What do our bodies need in order to achieve good health? The following sections will answer these questions as we review the different nutrients and their impact on body chemistry.

Fats

We all need fat in our diet, but the amount of the fat we consume must be low. Excess fat and the wrong types of fat are among the main causes of poor nutrition and headaches. The Loma Linda University study described in Chapter 2 plainly demonstrates that a low-fat diet can alleviate or even eliminate chronic headaches.

Furthermore, the type of fat you consume plays a significant role in good nutrition. There are three main types of fat—*saturated, polyunsaturated,* and *monounsaturated.* Saturated fat is found mostly in animal products, both meat and dairy, and in a few vegetable products, such as coconut oil and palm oil. High amounts of saturated fat in the diet can easily bring on a headache. How? Saturated fat increases levels of blood fat, including cholesterol, which promotes platelet clustering. This in turn reduces levels of serotonin. And as we saw in the Loma Linda study, decreased levels of serotonin cause the blood vessels to dilate, which usually precedes a headache.

The other types of fat are mostly of vegetable origin and are better for your health than saturated fat. The two most important fats are *omega-3* and *omega-6*. From a headache perspective, it is important to give preference to foods rich in omega-3, such as flaxseed oil, canola oil, soybeans, walnuts, and fish. Why? Omega-3 fats inhibit platelet clustering, while omega-6 fats promote platelet clustering. Reduced platelet clustering prevents the depletion of serotonin in the body. Excess amounts of omega-6 fats also increase levels of prostaglandins, some of which cause blood vessels to dilate. The ratio of omega-6 to omega-3 fats in your diet should be about five to one.

In addition to decreasing levels of serotonin, high-fat diets are largely responsible for obesity and chronic disorders such as hypercholesterolemia, hyperinsulinemia, and insulin resistance, which may cause headaches. The problem with high fat intake is that fat contains more than *twice* the calories than carbohydrates or proteins; there are nine calories for each gram of fat versus four calories for each gram of carbohydrate or protein. Worse yet, the body can easily store extra calories from dietary fat in the form of body fat. In one scientific study, researchers gave a group of subjects a 2,000-calorie meal in the form of carbohydrates. Only about 20 calories were converted and stored as body fat. Researchers then gave a second group of subjects a meal that contained 1,000 calories of fat more than they required. Nearly all the consumed fat was stored as body fat. And since stored fat causes high levels of blood fat and headaches, we can conclude that eating less fat and eating the right type of fat are crucial factors in headache prevention.

Carbohydrates

There are two types of carbohydrates—simple and complex. The first group includes the three simplest forms of sugar—glucose, fructose, and *galactose*. It also includes sucrose, or refined white sugar, which is the most common form of sugar. Simple carbohydrates occur naturally in many types of foods. The problem is that most refined or processed foods have a substantially higher percentage of simple carbohydrates than do nonrefined foods. This is because processing adds simple sugars to foods and removes many natural components that are beneficial to health. For example, white flour lacks many of the fibers, vitamins, and minerals that occur naturally in wheat because the refining process removes these elements. Canned fruits often contain large amounts of simple sugars, which alters the natural balance between simple and complex carbohydrates. If these fruits have been peeled or otherwise modified, they may have lost many of their fibers, vitamins, and minerals.

Complex carbohydrates include a wide range of starches, which are digestible, and dietary fibers, which pass through the body undigested. The best sources of complex carbohydrates are unprocessed fruits, grains, legumes, and vegetables. And although cooking and freezing do not significantly change the composition and health benefits of complex carbohydrates, they are best eaten raw.

To prevent headaches, you should replace the simple carbohydrates in your diet with complex carbohydrates. There are several reasons for this. First, refined sugars, such as those contained in soft drinks and candy, are easily digested, and they quickly raise blood-sugar levels. As explained in Chapter 2, this burst of energy releases too much insulin into the bloodstream, which results in a state of low blood sugar. So the body is forced to increase its blood-fat levels in order to provide adequate energy. The result is often a depletion of serotonin levels and the onset of a headache. Furthermore, if the excess energy produced by high-sugar foods is not expended by physical activity, it will be transformed into body fat.

The second reason for choosing complex carbohydrates over refined sugars is that headaches are frequently accompanied by changes in emotional state, including feelings of depression or anxiety. Such changes are caused by low levels of serotonin. Simple carbohydrates temporarily increase the amount of serotonin in the brain, causing a brief state of elation or well-being. But this increase is quickly followed by a reduction in serotonin, which signals a state of hunger and may cause a negative emotional response. If you respond by eating another high-sugar snack, the cycle is repeated. The situation is further exacerbated if the snack also contains a lot of fat, which only speeds up the degradation of serotonin. In contrast, a snack of complex carbohydrates increases levels of serotonin, but it will not trigger its rapid depletion.

The third reason for choosing foods rich in complex carbohydrates is that they contain a significant amount of dietary fibers. These indigestible particles are in all plant foods. They add volume to food, which makes it more filling without adding fat or any other calories. Fibers are beneficial in several important ways. First, some types of fibers, called *soluble* fibers, absorb water, thus further increasing the food volume and changing the ratios of fat to complex carbohydrates. Some fibers even lower levels of fat, notably cholesterol, in the blood. Fibers also slow the absorption of sugar and other nutrients, and therefore control the highs and lows in the levels of blood sugar that cause hypoglycemia, high blood fat, and headaches. Finally, fibers speed up the passage of food through the intestines, which automatically reduces the amount of calories extracted from the food. This helps prevent obesity and provides other health benefits.

The fourth reason for choosing foods rich in complex

carbohydrates is that these foods contain many different vitamins and minerals that play an important role in preventing headaches.

Proteins

Protein is an organic compound essential to sustain life. It contributes to essential body functions, including fluid balance, blood clotting, hormone and enzyme production, cell repair, immune functions, and metabolism. Protein is found in meats, dairy products, and a large variety of legumes, nuts, seeds, grains, and meat alternatives. From the perspective of relieving headaches, proteins of plant origin are preferable to proteins derived from animal products. Why? These foods provide protein in combination with carbohydrates, which help elevate levels of tryptophan in the body. Remember that tryptophan is essential for the production of serotonin in the brain. The amount of tryptophan that reaches the brain depends on its concentration in the blood and on the amount of other compounds in the body, such as carbohydrates. Thus, consuming protein in the form of legumes, nuts, seeds, grains, or meat alternatives greatly improves the absorption of tryptophan. This in turn produces more serotonin and helps prevent headaches.

Some plant foods—for example, avocados, nuts, and seeds—also contain considerable amounts of fat. Thus, they should be eaten in moderation. However, for headache prevention, this type of fat is still preferable to animal fat.

Another reason for limiting our intake of animal protein is that it is highly concentrated, and for this reason, it is easily consumed in excessive amounts. Too much protein can contribute to the occurrence of headaches. How? The digestive process breaks protein down into simpler compounds called *amino acids*. Amino acids are the building blocks of all cells and are used mainly for growth. But excess protein in the body can be turned into fat. In short, large amounts of animal protein are likely to increase levels of blood fat, which increases platelet clustering, decreases serotonin levels, and leads to headache.

Water

Water is the basic element of all tissues and fluids that make up the human body, and it is a major component of all foods. Many foods, for example, lettuce and melon, are over 90-percent water; and even foods that look dry, such as nuts or seeds, have some water content. Despite this, your body needs additional water for proper functioning. The amount of water required depends on your level of physical activity and your diet.

Water is particularly important to the digestive process. You need significant amounts of water to soften food in the stomach and break it down so that nutrients can pass into the bloodstream. Digestion changes the flow properties of blood. Before a meal, blood generally flows rapidly through all blood vessels. After a meal, especially one that is high in fat, blood flow comes to a relative crawl. Fat particles carried by the bloodstream are literally forced through the blood vessels. The result of this traffic jam is an increase in platelet clustering, which lowers serotonin levels and causes headaches.

Consuming significant amounts of liquids throughout the day, especially during meals, can improve this situation. Liquid dilutes the food and decreases the concentration of fats and other nutrients in the blood, making it flow more smoothly and preventing platelet damage. While the main ingredient in all beverages is water, plain water is still your best choice. Why? Other beverages may contain caffeine, alcohol, carbonation, sugar, and/or many chemicals that your body can certainly do without. Just read the list of ingredients on any can of diet soft drink. You may think twice before you take another sip.

Vitamins and Minerals

Vitamins and minerals facilitate different biochemical reactions, promote cell development, and improve the immune system. They occur naturally in foods rich in complex carbohydrates, especially fruits and vegetables. Unlike fats, carbohydrates, and proteins, only small quantities of vitamins and minerals are needed. However, their absence can have very serious consequences. Low levels of several vitamins and minerals may cause headaches because they influence levels of serotonin in the body. One of the most important is vitamin B_6, or *pyridoxine*, which helps produce serotonin from the amino acid tryptophan. Another important vitamin, vitamin B_3, or *niacin*, helps lower blood fat. Vitamin B_2, or *riboflavin*, is essential for the functioning of vitamins B_6 and B_3. Vitamin C is also necessary for the production of serotonin, and vitamin A helps decrease the levels of blood fat. Thus, adequate levels of all of these vitamins are important in preventing headaches.

Magnesium is the most important mineral in terms of headache prevention because it helps maintain the integrity of the blood vessels. Several scientific studies have shown that boosting levels of magnesium is very beneficial in alleviating headaches; and eating magnesium-rich foods such as tofu, soybeans, and spinach can do this. In fact, a well-balanced diet usually provides an adequate amount of vitamins and minerals. Nevertheless, additional vitamins and minerals in the form of supplements may also be useful, especially during the transition period when adapting to a new eating pattern.

Chemicals

Researchers have conducted many studies to identify specific nutrients or chemical substances that can cause headaches. The most commonly cited headache triggers are tyramine, found in red wines and cheese; *monosodium glu-*

tamate, or MSG, used as a flavor enhancer in many Chinese dishes and processed foods; *sodium nitrate,* found in cured meats; and *phenylethylamine.* In fact, there is some scientific evidence of a connection between these chemicals and headaches, but the evidence is not conclusive. A case in point is tyramine—one of the most widely cited headache triggers. Foods containing high levels of tyramine have indeed been shown to cause headaches; but foods high in tyramine, for example cheese, are also very high in fat. Furthermore, when tyramine was administered by itself to subjects in controlled experiments, the link to headache became very weak. This suggests that tyramine itself may not be a significant headache trigger. We can draw a similar conclusion about sodium nitrate and MSG, which are generally found in high-fat foods. Thus, the best approach to a healthy diet is to develop eating habits that keep the basic nutrients—fats, carbohydrates, proteins, water, vitamins, and minerals—in a natural balance.

WHY OUR DIETS ARE POOR

Animals in the wild do not consume foods that are bad for their health. Why is it that we humans knowingly and willingly expose ourselves to such a risk? Part of the answer may lie in our ingenuity, which has permitted us to alter our food supply and interfere with the healthy functioning of our bodies. The body needs all the basic nutrients to function properly, and for this reason, it has developed preferences for foods that contain the highest concentrations of these nutrients.

Since our early ancestors evolved in an environment where finding adequate amounts of fat was a challenge, we naturally prefer fatty foods. We also prefer sweet and salty tastes because in nature these tastes indicate the presence of carbohydrates, vitamins, and minerals—all of which are essential for survival. Memory also plays an important role in the foods we eat. Once we consume a food that has any nutritional value, the brain memorizes the food and tells us to search for it when we are hungry. This is part of our natural survival instinct. However, in our society, it is too easy to find any type of food any time we desire it.

In addition to having an overabundance of food, we are also able to alter foods by extracting nutrients from them, such as sugar and fat. These nutrients can then be combined to produce an almost limitless assortment of new foods containing unnaturally high ratios of certain nutrients. For example, margarine is made from oils using a process called *hydrogenation*. This greatly reduces omega-3 fats and increases saturated fats in the oils. White flour is made by milling grains and removing the surrounding shells—that is, the fibers. Chocolate and other rich sweets are examples of manufactured foods that combine fat and refined sugar, neither of which occur freely in nature.

The main problem with refined foods is that it is easy to eat too much of them. This is because the human body does not have a built-in satiation mechanism to signal that it is time to stop eating them. Even worse are foods that do not occur in nature at all, such as synthetic fats, which our bodies cannot recognize as harmful. If we restrict our intake of refined and processed foods, we can dramatically decrease the risk of becoming obese or developing other health problems, including headaches.

WHY SPECIAL DIETS DON'T WORK

People go on special diets with the hope of improving their health or their appearance. Although the two goals are frequently connected, the most common diets in our society are weight-loss diets. Not surprisingly, many books, magazines, and other outlets publish all sorts of weight-loss diets. Most promise unrealistic results, and in the end, they only create frustration.

The main reason most weight-loss diets do not work is that they impose temporary restrictions on certain types of foods. This causes feelings of deprivation, which only intensify the desire for the forbidden foods. Not surprisingly, at the end of a diet period, the suppressed desires often take over, and the dieter regains all or more of his initial weight.

The second major reason that diets fail is that rapid weight loss cannot be sustained for very long. Contrary to the promises of many weight-loss diets, it is impossible to lose a significant amount of fat within a few weeks. In addition, if the weight comes off too quickly, the metabolism slows considerably in an effort to save itself from starvation. The inability to lose weight quickly and the frustrations produced by food deprivation generally break the spirit and determination of all but the strongest person. A reasonable rate of weight loss that can be sustained over a long period is about one to two pounds per week.

Some diets fail simply because they do not offer a variety of foods. People can easily develop an aversion to an extremely limited set of food choices, which gives them a reason to give up. Lack of variety can also result in inadequate levels of important vitamins, minerals, and other nutrients. The only healthy approach to improving nutrition is to modify your eating habits gradually as you develop the taste for new, healthier foods. As long as you perceive food deprivation, you will not be able to sustain the changes for long.

GUIDELINES FOR GOOD NUTRITION

Since special diets do not work, is there anything we can do to change our eating habits for the better? Or will we forever have to make the difficult choice between healthy foods and foods we like to eat? Yes, we can change our eating habits, and we can gradually change our taste for different foods.

A good way to visualize your long-term nutritional goals is to stack the different food groups in a "food pyramid" like the one in Figure 3.1 on page 56. Each layer of the Food Pyramid represents a basic food group, and the number of servings indicates how much or how little of these

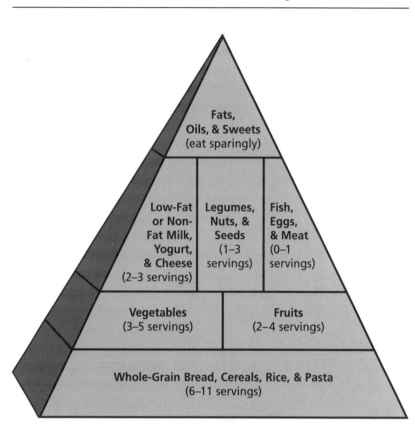

Figure 3.1. Food Pyramid

sorts of foods should be consumed each day. I recommend this particular Food Pyramid—which is based on the one published by the United States Department of Agriculture—for the most effective headache prevention.

Make Healthful Food Choices

The Food Pyramid represents basic principles of healthy nutrition in the form of a visual guideline. Unfortunately, the eating habits of many people show a different picture—a pyramid in which fats, oils, and sweets make up the largest volume, while sources of complex carbohydrates are underrepresented. Remember that your long-term goal is not to eliminate particular foods from your diet, but to re-arrange the contents of your pyramid so that its ratios approach those of the Food Pyramid.

How you shape your own pyramid depends largely on two things—the way you cook and the restaurants you frequent. When you prepare most of your meals yourself, it is much easier to control the ratios of the different types of foods. The most important factors to consider are the amounts and types of fat you use. Some traditional recipes are loaded with fat, but it is not difficult to prepare exquisite tasting meals using little or no fat. To learn the necessary techniques and to get some fresh ideas, visit your local bookstore and pick up a few books on low-fat cooking. Some great selections are listed at the back of this book in the Recommended Readings section. You may also wish to explore the many ethnic cookbooks that offer wonderful low-fat recipes. In addition, there are some excellent vegetarian cookbooks; but keep in mind that vegetarian does not necessarily mean low fat. You must still pay attention to the shape of your food pyramid as the most important long-term goal.

If you rely on restaurants for many of your meals, controlling the amounts and ratios of the basic food types can be a challenge. However, the strategies presented in this chapter are designed to help you gradually introduce changes toward a healthier way of eating. Although our food preferences are shaped most strongly in childhood, they continue developing throughout our lives. We are able to acquire a taste for new foods, and we are able to reduce our desire for certain foods.

It is ironic that many people avoid the healthiest foods because of the way they may feel after eating them. A very common complaint is that fresh fruit and vegetables cause digestive problems such as heartburn, indigestion, diarrhea, or gas. The truth of the matter is that these discomforts are caused by the fatty and unbalanced food in your diet. When you eat a lot of fatty foods every day for many years, your digestive system learns to expect them with each meal, and it adapts by producing extra stomach juices and fluids. If you suddenly begin to eat lots of fruits and vegetables, the increase may trigger various discomforts. Nevertheless, you can easily avoid these problems by introducing new foods slowly.

Choose Whole-Grain Products

The largest portion of your daily nutrition should come from complex carbohydrates in the form of breads, cereals, rice, and pasta. However, it is very important to choose whole-grain products because the grains are close to their natural state. This guarantees an adequate supply of complex carbohydrates, including fibers, minerals, vitamins, and other important substances.

A helpful strategy to increase your intake of complex carbohydrates and displace fat in your diet is to learn to enjoy simple foods. In the quest to satisfy our palate with fancy foods, we sometimes forget how good some basic foods can taste. When did you last eat bread with nothing on it? Try it, and you may be surprised. Many supermarkets and specialty stores offer a large selection of tasty breads and other wholesome baked goods. Choose whole-grain, enriched breads. Or, better yet, find a bakery that bakes crispy or firm dark crusty bread daily.

You can enjoy many other basic foods that are rich in complex carbohydrates. For example, try whole-grain pasta, rice, and various beans. Good pasta with fresh tomatoes and garlic does not have to float in butter or cream sauce to taste great. You may be surprised to find that good freshly cooked rice tastes wonderful by itself or with just a touch of soy sauce or other seasoning. The same goes for beans and lentils—a can of low-fat or nonfat baked beans with bread is a great alternative to burgers and fries. The complex carbohydrates in these dishes will reduce your blood-fat levels and provide important vitamins and minerals to help prevent headaches.

Choose Fruits and Vegetables

Gradually replacing dietary fat with a variety of fruits and vegetables has several major benefits. Most fruits and vegetables are a major source of complex carbohydrates, and they are the most important sources of vitamins and minerals. For the best results in headache prevention, I suggest that you eat five servings of vegetables and four servings of fruits every day. Fruits and vegetables are also beneficial to digestion. They contain a high percentage of water, lots of fiber, and usually almost no fat. In addition, the natural juices contained in fruits and vegetables aid the body in the digestion of fat.

Limit Protein

Protein is essential for good health, but you do not need it in large amounts. The recommended daily amount of protein is two to three servings. The USDA Food Pyramid recommends two to three servings of meat, poultry, fish, dry beans, eggs, and nuts. Nevertheless, combining these different types of foods in one group while excluding others such as lentils, peas, and meat alternatives may not be the best choice for headache prevention. Therefore, the Food Pyramid in Figure 3.1 creates two separate groups. The first includes legumes in general—pinto beans, black beans, white beans, navy beans, soybeans, chick peas, lentils, green peas, peanuts, and many others. This food group also includes a variety of nuts, seeds, and soybean products, notably tofu and different meat alternatives. The second group contains meats, fish, and eggs. These provide animal proteins, but also significant amounts of animal fat. For effective headache prevention, they should be eaten in small quantities. There is no need to be concerned about a lack of protein as long as you increase the amounts of breads, rice, pasta, legumes, and other foods as recommended.

Limit Fat Intake

The tip of the Food Pyramid is made up of fats, oils, and

sweets, which you should use sparingly. The best type of fat is of vegetable origin. Olive oil is a great choice, but you must also include fats that contain sufficient amounts of omega-3. The total amount of fat consumed is very important. A very conservative recommendation by the Food and Nutrition Board Committee is that no more than 30 percent of calories come from fat. The American Heart Association recommends that between 15 and 20 percent of calories come from fat. For effective headache prevention, I recommend that you gradually reduce you fat intake to the 15- to 20-percent range.

What does this mean in terms of fat grams? The answer depends on the number of calories you should be eating; and this is determined by factors such as your weight, age, gender, activity level, and metabolism. However, to give you an approximate recommendation, the range for the average adult should be between 25 and 55 grams of fat per day. That is, a person who weighs about 150 pounds, maintains at least some level of physical activity, and is not overweight or suffering from any chronic disorders should aim for no more than 40 grams of fat per day.

How can you determine the number of fat grams you consume? There are two main sources of information. Most packaged foods have food labels that list the total amount of fat per serving and the number of servings contained in the package. When a product does not have a food label or when you dine out, you will have to consult a "fat finder." These booklets, which are available in most bookstores, list the amount of fat in a great variety of foods. Buy the smallest one and carry it with you wherever you go. Before buying or eating any foods, consult it to find out how much fat you are about to consume.

This may sound like a lot of work, but it really is not. In fact, you may enjoy doing this sort of detective work, and you will be surprised by the amount of fat you generally consume. When you consider that a slice of cheesecake may have as many as 60 grams of fat, and a cheeseburger with fries may contain 50 to 80 grams of fat, you can see how easy it is to eat many times the recommended amount of fat. With time, you will be able to guess the amount of fat in most common foods, and maintaining the recommended amount will become more or less automatic.

If you sometimes exceed the recommended amount, don't get discouraged. People are not robots. Many circumstances influence our actions. It is perfectly normal to let go occasionally. Instead of blaming yourself, drink a lot of water and increase your intake of complex carbohydrates the following day to make up for your relapse. Don't give up.

One of the most important things to remember is that reducing your fat intake should be done very gradually over a period of several weeks, or even months if your current fat intake is very high. It is quite possible that you will not have to reduce your fat intake to the lowest level recommended. You may realize that even a modest decrease in fat consumption can prevent your headaches. By slowly limiting your normal intake of fatty foods and substituting them with more nutritious, less fatty foods, you will discover how easy it is to develop a taste for good nutrition.

Increase Water Intake

Increasing the amount of water you drink on a daily basis is very important for preventing headaches. You should get into the habit of drinking water throughout the day. Drink one glass of water when you get up in the morning. During the night, you lose quite a bit of water, and it is important to restore the balance and get your digestive system going. The water will also calm your hunger. This way, when you have breakfast, you will be able to think more clearly about what you should eat, and you will be less likely to reach for the easiest, and perhaps most unhealthy, thing you happen to see.

You should also get in the habit of having a glass of water before, during, and after your meals. But you must develop this habit gradually as you decrease your intake of fat. In fact, if you drink water with very fatty foods, the water makes it more difficult for the body to digest them. However, digestion can be improved by decreasing the amount of fat in your diet. If you always associate water with eating, you will be less likely to forget to drink it—you will have a set schedule for it at least three times a day.

You should also keep a bottle of water with you at all times so you can have a drink any time you feel even a hint of thirst. If you have water nearby, you can quench your thirst before drinking a carbonated or caffeinated beverage. Water is truly the best and most natural thirst quencher!

STAYING ON TRACK

You know that in order to prevent headaches, you must improve your eating habits. We have given you a basic idea of what you should be eating; but what can you do to make sure that you stay on track? It is relatively easy to start a program of nutritious eating, but following it can be a difficult challenge. The strategies discussed in the following sections will help you maintain your new healthful diet.

Begin Slowly

Do not expect to change your eating habits overnight. It takes time to develop a taste for new, healthier types of food. If you attempt to break your bad habits by force, your body will rebel, and you will quickly end up where you started. The good news is that people rarely go from good to bad in terms of their nutrition. At a young age, living on hamburgers and milkshakes seems like the most natural thing to do; but with advancing age, our sense of invincibility wanes, and we become more health-conscious.

Expect to go through several stages as you begin to think about a healthier diet. The earliest stage of change is *denial*—you feel that your eating habits are perfectly fine, and there is no need to do anything. But at some point, you will reach the stage of *contemplation,* when you begin to admit that you must make some changes in your diet. Once you have decided to do this, you are ready to act. The most critical phase comes after your initial action—you must *sustain* the effort, which generally leads to doubts and relapses.

Remember that a specific diet always has a beginning and an end. It is usually perceived as a period of suffering and self-sacrifice, and so it leads to an even greater desire for the forbidden foods. However, when you slowly add more complex carbohydrates to your diet and decrease your intake of fatty foods, there are no specific limitations or forbidden foods. It is a slow process, but it will eventually free you from the desire for unhealthy foods. You will also find yourself liking different types of food. Since you can still eat the foods you are used to, you won't experience the cravings you normally do during a diet, and at the same time, you will be introduced to new foods and eating habits. You will naturally decrease your caloric intake due to changes in your eating habits. You will start feeling great and have more energy. And you will no longer have your headaches.

Eat Slowly

When you eat your food too quickly, you do not give yourself time to enjoy it, and you can actually feel deprived after eating a meal. Eating slowly will give you the time to enjoy what you are eating. Many people admire France for its cuisine, which is based on rich creamy sauces, butter, cheeses, and delicious sweets. Yet, obesity and eating disorders are much less of a problem in France than in the United States. The key is the amount of food consumed per unit of time. A simple meal in France can easily take two hours, and a ten-course dinner does not necessarily imply overeating—on the contrary. A course may consist of three small mushrooms, yet a Frenchman can spend fifteen minutes enjoying it. If you like French or other high-calorie cooking—and there is nothing wrong with that as long as you only eat it occasionally—you must learn to reduce your portions and eat very slowly.

There are some physiological reasons that you should eat slowly. Remember that it takes time for your digestive system to recognize food intake. The stomach expands as it receives food, and at some point, it starts sending messages to the brain that it has had enough. If you eat too quickly, you will outpace your digestive system and eat too much food before it can signal that you are full. By slowing down, you will have better control over how much you eat and what you eat.

Reorder Your Plate

To achieve balanced nutrition, use the Food Pyramid as your guide when filling your plate—the higher an item is located on the pyramid, the smaller its amount should be. This strategy is especially useful in a buffet-style situation, where you have a choice of many tempting foods. Have a glass of water, and then fill your plate with salad, vegetables, and other foods rich in complex carbohydrates. But promise yourself that you will come back and enjoy some of the other foods you like to eat. In the meantime, the complex carbohydrates will fill you up physically and psychologically, and you will not be so tempted by foods that may not be good for you. By reordering your plate in this way, you will increase the level of serotonin in your body. This signals your brain that you are satisfied, and satisfaction early in the meal helps you reduce the total amount of food you eat.

When you get cravings for cookies, ice cream, or other sweets, apply the same strategy. Instead of automatically thinking, "I mustn't eat these!" make it a rule to drink a glass of water and eat some complex carbohydrates first—a piece of fruit or vegetable, for example. This will satisfy your body's need to increase its serotonin levels. The next step is to satisfy your psychological need for the "forbidden food," which is now a much simpler task. In fact, when you follow this method, there are no forbidden foods; there are only delays in eating them, or perhaps a change of mind. After a few weeks, you will notice that your body will start demanding more of the complex carbohydrates, and—unbelievable as it may sound—you will begin to lose interest in the forbidden foods.

Eat Regularly

Another important rule is to eat regularly, because skipping meals and fasting are potent headache triggers. However, if you get hungry during the day and do not satisfy your hunger, blood fat increases and serotonin continues to drop until a headache develops. You need a snack. Snacking on sugary, high-fat foods can make the problem even worse. The sugar boost causes a temporary state of satisfaction, but the fat quickly erodes serotonin to an even lower level, and this results in more feelings of hunger and headaches. The only good snacks are complex carbohydrates, preferably from fruits or vegetables. An apple, a carrot, or a banana will help you get through until your next meal by supplying necessary energy and filling your stomach—without the fat. Plus complex carbohydrates help increase the levels of serotonin due to the higher amounts of vitamin B_6.

Reduce Caffeine

Many people use a cup of coffee or some other caffeinated beverage as a quick snack. In fact, some of my headache patients used to drink as many as ten to twelve cups of coffee a day. When they came in for a headache consultation, they made it very clear that if I were to tell them to stop drinking coffee they would leave. Some habits and addictions are so powerful that even the thought of having to break them is frightening. The key to reducing caffeine is not to eliminate coffee from your diet, but to learn to substitute it with decaffeinated coffee or preferably water. For example, try to drink a glass of water before having a cup of coffee. If the water quenches your thirst, you may find that you do not even want the coffee. At the very least, the water will dilute the general effect of the coffee on your body.

Another highly recommended approach to reducing caffeine is to drink tea. There are many varieties of teas as well as ways of preparing them. Some can be just as strong and aromatic as good coffee, and they can be taken with milk, just like coffee; others are soothing and healing. Pick up a book on teas and give yourself a basic education in the art of preparing and enjoying tea. Better yet, ask someone from Great Britain, India, the Middle East, Japan, China, or any other place where tea is a daily affair. You may get not only advice on tea, but also a lecture on an entirely different philosophy of life.

Don't Let Hunger Influence Your Actions

Hunger is a powerful manipulator, and it can significantly distort your perceptions and sense of reason. You should avoid situations where you are obliged to make decisions about food when you are hungry. This applies especially to food shopping. When you are hungry, almost anything looks enticing, and you will most likely end up with more than you really need. You might also be tempted to buy the types of food you would normally avoid. You can minimize this risk by shopping only after a meal.

A more challenging situation is ordering food in a restaurant. Drinking a glass of water or eating a piece of fruit shortly before looking at the menu will help restore your sense of reality. It is a good idea to avoid appetizers that are loaded with fat. Buffet-style restaurants present a special challenge due to the large variety and supply of food. If you cannot avoid them, it is crucial that you remember to order your plate using the Food Pyramid as a guide and to eat slowly. Remember that the first plate is the most critical. If you stack it with foods rich in complex carbohydrates on your first pass, you may not even want to go back for a refill.

Pay Attention to Your Food

A good way to stay on track is to take the time to enjoy your meals. For example, do not eat while you are concentrating on some other task, especially when you are hungry. Always take time to eat before starting your task, and try to keep the two activities separate. And never keep a cache of snacks around when you are immersed in solving a problem. You could end up consuming a lot of food without even noticing it.

Business or professional meetings can sometimes be a problem. In most routine situations, you can enjoy your food while talking about business-related matters. Casual talking does not interfere with eating. On the contrary, it will slow you down and stop you from gulping your food. However, if the purpose of your meeting is to make an important presentation, lead a discussion, make a sale, or any other situation that requires your full attention, you will not be able to think about what you are eating. In such a situation, order the simplest possible food—a small salad or a bowl of soup—and concentrate on the task at hand. Anything else is a waste of money, since you will not even know what you are eating. Worse yet, you run the risk of eating too much, and your dissatisfaction will lead to another big meal at dinner. Remember the adage, "Don't mix business with pleasure"—if the focus on business is crucial, make it a simple meal.

CONCLUSION

A diet low in fat, refined sugar, and processed food, and high in complex carbohydrates is one of the most important steps in preventing headaches. Now that you have learned how to develop a taste for foods that will help you eliminate headaches, you are ready to explore the importance of regular physical activity and exercise on your body's biochemistry and its influence on headaches. The next chapter will start you on the second phase of my program.

CHAPTER 4

Physical Activity
and Headache

Lack of activity destroys the good condition of
every human being,
while movement and methodical exercise save
and preserve it.

—Plato

There is no doubt that regular physical activity can lower the incidence of headaches. In fact, regular physical activity is a powerful medicine quite unlike any pain medication. But although most people are aware that exercise is beneficial, they don't always know how to make it part of their lives. Together with improved nutrition, it forms a major component of my headache prevention and treatment program. However, I will not ask you to join an aerobics class or jog five miles every morning. My goal is to help you develop a taste for more physical activity so that you learn to enjoy it. Before presenting the approach and specific strategies to achieve the seemingly impossible, we must first understand the basic impact of physical activity on headaches and health in general.

PHYSICAL ACTIVITY AND BODY CHEMISTRY

Any form of physical activity has a direct impact on the

functioning of the body because it triggers different bio-chemical processes. Many of these processes can prevent headaches, but others can cause them. For this reason, it is important to understand what types and levels of exercise are appropriate for headache prevention. Regular activity also tends to improve the physical fitness of the body over time. In addition, this positive aspect plays an enormous role in preventing headaches and other chronic diseases.

Burning Fat

We have already seen that fat, both in the bloodstream and deposited as body tissue, is one of the main causes of head-aches. Physical activity directly reduces fat in the blood-stream, and depending on a number of other circumstances, it may reduce fat deposits and increase muscle tissue. Let us examine some of the biochemical processes that are influenced by exercise.

The human body needs energy to power its muscles, to perform various biochemical functions, and to generate heat. Our main sources of energy are carbohydrates and fats; and although both sources are important, each plays a very different role. It is relatively easy for the body to con-vert carbohydrates into energy. At the start of any activity, the necessary energy comes primarily from carbohydrates—that is, blood sugar and sugar stored in muscle cells. This form of energy is called *anaerobic* because it can be released without the use of oxygen. But the body's sugar reserves are quickly depleted during physical activity, and the body starts using blood fat for energy. This requires oxygen, and the resulting energy is called *aerobic*.

Strenuous exercise burns carbohydrates very rapidly. After only two minutes of such an activity, carbohydrates supply half the energy and fats supply half the energy. Ten minutes later, fats supply most of the energy. Light or mod-erate activity takes longer to reach the fat-burning stage be-cause stored sugar in the body continues to supply energy for a longer period. Consequently, the duration of physical activity is the most important factor in reducing blood fat and body fat.

When blood sugar and blood fat are not used for energy, they are converted into body fat and stored. Over time, this leads to an unhealthy ratio of body fat to muscle tissue, which brings about two important changes in the body's metabolism that can contribute to headaches. First, the unhealthy ratio of muscle tissue to fat tissue decreases the body's resting metabolism—the amount of energy needed when the body is not performing any physical activity. Why? Fat tissue requires less energy than muscle tissue. Second, a sedentary body has a much lower capacity to clear fat from the blood. In fact, studies have shown that athletes can eliminate fat from blood after a meal twice as fast as people who lead sedentary lifestyles.

Releasing Hormones

Physical activity has a major impact on the body's hormones, which regulate many functions of the body. Hormones generally keep the various biochemical processes in balance; that is, in a stable, steady state commonly referred to as homeostasis. From the headache perspective, the most important hormones are those that help the body use fat as a source of energy. They include *epinephrine, glucagon,* and the growth hormone *somatotropin.* Levels of these hormones increase with physical activity, which helps convert body fat into blood fat for immediate use as energy. Glucagon also increases the production of blood sugar in the liver, which serves as an additional energy source to cope with the increased physical activity.

While a healthy level of exercise is highly beneficial in preventing headaches, excessive physical activity can also trigger headaches. How? Over-exercising causes the release of disproportionate amounts of the above three hormones, which results in the production of too much blood fat. This increases platelet clustering, decreases serotonin, and leads to vasodilatation and headache. The situation is further exacerbated by the release of prostaglandins, which cause more platelet clustering and contribute to the degradation of serotonin.

Insulin, whose main function is to regulate levels of blood sugar, is another important hormone affected by exercise. Physical activity has an insulin-like effect in that it improves the body's ability to use blood sugar. Therefore, the body needs less insulin to process blood sugar. In the end, this reduces the risk of developing certain chronic conditions that cause headaches. Two of these conditions, hyperinsulinemia and insulin resistance are discussed in Chapter 2.

Finally, physical activity releases several hormones into the bloodstream that increase the threshold of pain perception and promote a state of well-being. One of the best known of these hormones, *beta-endorphin*, is released during long-duration exercise and acts as a natural pain reliever.

Improving Blood Flow

Two of the most important functions of blood are to transport oxygen and nutrients throughout the body and to carry away the various byproducts of the biochemical processes. The amount of blood that flows to different parts of the body varies in accordance with the type and level of physical activity. At rest, especially after a meal, much of the blood is diverted to the digestive organs, and muscles receive only about 20 percent of the blood flow. Exercise or any other physical activity changes this distribution dramatically. For example, light exercise such as walking increases blood flow to muscles to about 50 percent of total blood flow, but heavy exercise can increase blood flow to over 80 percent.

The brain is of particular interest when examining headache because it requires a constant supply of oxygen. Lack of oxygen automatically triggers a widening of the blood vessels in the brain to allow more blood to flow through them. In order to prevent this, more oxygen must be supplied to the brain. The best way to do this is by deep breathing and by increasing your level of physical activity. Any increase, even as simple as getting up from your chair and taking a walk, will increase your heart rate. As the heart beats faster, it pumps more blood through the body. At the same time, the blood vessels adjust their tension so they can transport blood to the parts of the body that need it most. The brain will then get its share of oxygen without having to widen the blood vessels.

Physical activity also restores blood circulation to skeletal muscles and gives them a chance to recover from fatigue. Skeletal muscles have two main functions. First, they enable the body to move. Second, they maintain body posture. Even when no part of the body is moving, a number of muscles are needed to keep the body in place. Thus, some parts of our bodies are working even when we are at rest. This applies especially to the neck and shoulder muscles, which support the head in its upright position. Given the considerable weight of the human head, two things are of importance—good posture and adequate physical activity. Good posture guarantees that your head is well balanced and that there is minimal strain on your support muscles. Physical activity ensures that your support muscles do not become tired. However, lack of exercise increases discomfort and muscle tenderness in the neck and shoulders. This can cause muscle contractions, which irritate nerve endings and may cause headaches. The best way to prevent this is to take regular breaks and do a few stretching exercises.

In addition to the short-term benefits of improved blood flow, exercise has major long-term benefits. First, increased blood flow through muscle tissues increases the utilization of fat as energy, which helps reduce body fat. Increased blood flow is also highly beneficial to the cardiovascular system. It gets the heart and blood vessels into better shape so that they can more readily and more easily respond to the demands of increased physical activity.

WHY WE LEAD SEDENTARY LIVES

Why is it that some people truly enjoy physical activity while others seem to do everything possible to avoid anything that cannot be done in a sitting position? One of the main reasons is that exercise and inactivity are habit-forming. Children naturally enjoy physical activity—playing ball, climbing trees and rocks, running, and physically challenging one another in all sorts of games. These are natural activities that help children develop their body coordination and strength and that help their bodies regulate many biochemical processes. Levels of physical activity tend to decrease with age, and some people begin to develop life-long habits of inactivity.

Many things contribute to inactivity, and some of these are a result of technological progress. Our earliest ancestors lived as hunters and gatherers, depending on nature and simple weapons for their survival, which required a lot of walking and other exercise. The development of agriculture made the food supply more predictable, and industrialization improved the efficiency with which food and other goods were produced. Food production still requires a significant amount of physical work, but the activity is frequently repetitive, and may lead to various chronic health problems that interfere with regular exercise and recreational activities. The development of computers, robots, and other forms of automation during the last few decades—the information and electronics age—has made it possible for many people to earn their livings without exerting themselves physically. For the first time in the history of civilization, it has become possible for many people to live their entire lives doing only a minimal amount of physical work. This luxury has further contributed to the development of sedentary lifestyles.

Although the shift from mostly physical to mostly mental work reduced the amount of physical activity performed on a daily basis, it did little to diminish the level of fatigue most people feel at the end of a working day. While they may not be exhausted physically, they still feel very tired and drained, and may find it difficult to start engaging in any form of physical exercise. What many people do not realize is that a short walk in the evening would provide them with much more energy than a passive form of relaxation, such as watching television.

Chronic health problems may also cause physical inactivity. An aching back or bad knees are common reasons for not exercising. Excess body weight and a resulting lack of self-esteem often discourage people. However, it is never too late to reverse your condition. Many chronic illnesses can be greatly alleviated, and sometimes even completely reversed, through appropriate lifestyle changes. It is up to you to take matters into your own hands and start repairing the damage of years of neglecting your body.

WHY SOME EXERCISE PROGRAMS DON'T WORK

Do the words, "You must exercise!" scare or depress you because you immediately imagine hours of running, workouts in the gym, and interruptions in your busy schedule? Do you think of exercise as an unpleasant necessity and use various excuses to get out of doing it whenever possible? There is a simple truth about physical activity—to do it regularly and to sustain it, you have to enjoy it. In a way, physical activity is the counterpart to eating—one supplies the calories while the other uses them up. But just as dieting may not work because it forbids you to eat certain foods, a prescribed exercise program may not work because it forces you to do something you resent. Forbidding and prescribing something are just two sides of the same coin.

This book is concerned with physical activity as a means of preventing headaches. The main objective is to reduce your amount of body fat and blood fat, and you can do this with regular physical activity. One of the main reasons for the failure of many exercise programs is that people choose activities they dislike. Furthermore, they often overwork themselves at the beginning. In an initial moment of excitement, it is very easy to overdo any new physical activity, which can leave your muscles feeling sore for days afterward.

To increase your physical activity and sustain it for the rest of your life, you must experience the benefits of that activity. Just as you can gradually develop a taste for different foods, you can also learn to enjoy physical activity. If you hate exercise, you may never reach the point where you look forward to going to the gym. Nevertheless, there are still plenty of physical activities you can learn to enjoy.

It is important to remember that increasing your activity is as important to your life as breathing. But the process must be slow, especially if you have led a sedentary life until this point. If you force yourself to go to the gym, you will go for one or two weeks and then find convincing excuses not to go. Even if you are certain that physical activity offers many benefits, joining a health club may not be the right first step. You will go to the gym when you are ready. Start by using the stairs instead of the elevator, and eventually you may work your way to the StairMaster at the gym.

TYPES OF PHYSICAL ACTIVITY

There are three main types of physical activity, or exercise—aerobic, anaerobic, and stretching—and each contributes in some way to the prevention of headaches. For the best results, you should perform all three types on a regular basis. Nevertheless, it is even more important that you enjoy what you are doing. With exercise, this is easy because there are many options.

Aerobic Exercises

Aerobic exercises are sustained exercises that rely primarily on oxygen and that strengthen the heart and lungs. Remember that at the start of any physical activity, much of the energy is derived from sugar. Sugar is delivered very rapidly, but since its reserves are limited, the energy does not last very long. To sustain an activity over longer a period, the body must switch to fat as its main energy source. With strenuous exercise, such as running, swimming, or aerobic dancing, this happens within a few minutes. Light or moderate activities, such as walking or bicycling at a leisurely pace, do not require as much energy. But they can be sustained and enjoyed for much longer periods, and this makes them the best forms of aerobic activities for headache prevention. Remember that it is not the difficulty of an activity that makes it aerobic, but its duration. All aerobic exercises are great fat burners and tension reducers. In addition, they strengthen the working muscles and the cardiovascular system, burn fat, and prevent the development of headaches.

Anaerobic Exercises

Anaerobic exercises are those that rely on immediate or short-term energy, called anaerobic energy. This is the form of energy derived from sugar and other chemicals stored in muscle cells and blood. Anaerobic energy is delivered much more rapidly than aerobic energy and its release requires no oxygen. Therefore, it is essential for activities that require fast movement, such as a high jump, a golf swing, or a sprint. Anaerobic energy is also essential for resistance exercises such as weightbearing and other muscle-strengthening exercises.

The main purpose of anaerobic exercises is to strengthen skeletal muscles and improve their ability to perform quick and powerful movements. The exercises complement aerobic activities, which rely on large skeletal muscles. Increasing muscle tissue, usually at the expense of excess fat tissue, also improves the percentage of body fat. While it may not decrease total body weight, it makes the body appear more athletic and, more important, it reduces the level of blood fat.

Stretching Exercises

Stretching exercises improve muscle tone and increase blood circulation. Their main purpose is to prevent cramping and stiffness of muscles, which lead to discomfort, pain, or injury. You should do some very simple forms of stretching several times a day as part of regular breaks from work or other activities. Stretching should also be included in your warm-up routine before any other form of exercise. This will gradually increase your heart rate and respiration, loosen your muscles and prepare them for activity by supplying them with blood and nutrients, and reduce the risk of injury. Stretching is also a good way to wind down an aerobic or muscle-strengthening exercise session as part of your cool-down routine to prevent soreness and stiffness.

GUIDELINES FOR PHYSICAL ACTIVITY

As already mentioned, one of the worst things you can do is begin an exercise program that you do not enjoy. But what if you simply don't enjoy any sort of physical activity? Is there any hope for you? The answer is yes. Just as you can gradually develop the taste for different foods, you can also learn to enjoy physical activity.

A good way to visualize your long-term exercise goal is to arrange your activities according to the Physical Activity Pyramid in Figure 4.1 on page 79. The positions of each layer indicate the relative importance of each type of activity and how much time it will require in your daily schedule. Figure 4.1, which is based on a similar one published in the *Health and Fitness Journal*, describes the physical activities I recommend for the most effective headache prevention.

Make Healthful Exercise Choices

The precise amount and type of activity needed each day varies from individual to individual. But everyone can find an activity that he or she likes or can learn to enjoy. When some people hear the word exercise, they immediately think of health clubs, gyms, or athletic tracks; but almost anything we do in a standing position is a physical activity. You may

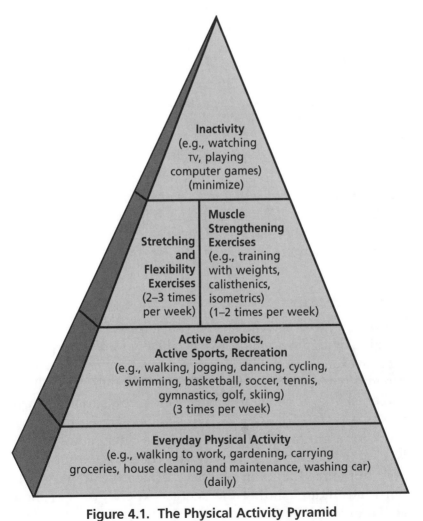

Figure 4.1. The Physical Activity Pyramid

never derive any pleasure from a game of tennis or an aerobic dance class; but you will probably enjoy activities such as gardening, walking in the park, or playing with your child or grandchild.

The Physical Activity Pyramid provides a visual guideline for the recommended levels and types of physical activities that you should aim for. For effective headache prevention, you need a combination of stretching, anaerobic, and aerobic activities. Just remember that exercise should not cause pain and that your way to a higher level of fitness must be gradual. Light or moderate exercise will have many more benefits than exhausting exercise. Moderate activity tends to decrease appetite, and it has a positive impact on your state of mind. In addition, regular light or moderate activity is relatively easy to sustain over time.

Include Aerobic Activities

Many people associate aerobics with a lot of vigorous jumping and running. However, it is not the intensity, but the duration of the activity that makes it aerobic. This is because the body needs sufficient time to reach the fat-using stage. Thus, a long walk is an aerobic activity, but a 100-yard dash is mostly anaerobic because it relies primarily on carbohydrates.

There are different forms of aerobic activities—*active aerobics, active sports,* and *active recreation.* Some of these are noncompetitive activities, such as aerobic dance or brisk walking or jogging, which are specifically for the purpose of aerobic exercise. Active sports and recreation include a wide range of competitive activities, such as tennis, basketball, soccer, skiing, rowing, and gymnastics. You should engage in some form of aerobic activity at least three times per week for a minimum of twenty minutes, depending on the level of the activity. The activity you choose is entirely up to you; but since the main objective of aerobic activity is to burn fat, understanding the energy expenditures of these activities will help you make the right choices.

Table 4.1 lists the number of calories expended after performing a given activity for one hour. The range of calories burned depends on how much a person weighs. The average weight for purposes of the table is between 125 and 215 pounds.

TABLE 4.1. CALORIE-BURNING EXERCISES	
Activity	**Calories Burned Per Hour**
Jogging at 6 mph	570–980
Cycling at 10 mph	570–980
Swimming (fast)	570–980
Basketball	462–810
Tennis	455–785
Aerobic dance (low impact)	285–490
Walking at 4 mph	260–440
Walking at 3.5 mph	228–390
Gymnastics	222–390
Volleyball	168–294

The exercises in Table 4.1 are arranged from the highest to lowest energy-expenditure values. It is not surprising that jogging, cycling, and swimming consume the most energy, followed closely by active sports such as basketball and tennis. It is interesting that aerobic dance, which seems to be quite challenging, ranks only slightly higher than walking. Furthermore, walking expends more energy per hour than gymnastics or many other competitive sports such as volleyball.

Given the above comparison, walking is perhaps the easiest form of aerobic exercise you can do. Since even our earliest ancestors had to walk considerable distances, the human body is well equipped for this activity. Walking is a low-impact activity with no negative side effects, and any age group can do it. It takes no special training or equipment. All you need are loose-fitting clothing and a good pair of walking shoes.

Before committing yourself to a specialized aerobic program or sport, you must consider the level of your everyday life activities. In many cases, these already include aerobic type activities, such as walking to work or school, taking care of the house or garden, and carrying groceries. Table 4.2 lists the energy expended after an hour of doing a typical household activity.

TABLE 4.2. CALORIE-BURNING ACTIVITIES	
Activity	**Calories Burned Per Hour**
Scrubbing floors	366–642
Gardening	303–528
Housecleaning	210–366
Window cleaning	198–348
Cooking	150–264

It is worth noting that many of these activities are more effective in burning calories than many specialized exercises, including aerobic dancing. However, aerobic exercises are essential to the reduction of body fat and blood fat, and all activities can help prevent headaches.

Include Muscle-Fitness Exercises

Muscle-fitness exercises work to increase or maintain muscle strength and endurance. This means that they increase the volume of muscle tissue and eliminate excess fat tissue. These activities rely mostly on anaerobic energy, but they still burn a significant number of calories. For example, training with weights will consume between 340 and 590 calories per hour.

There are several ways to perform muscle-strengthening exercises. The most common is to use weights for resistance. These can be free weights, such as dumbbells or barbells, or they can be weight-training machines, which are available in health clubs and gyms. If you do not have weights, you can start by using common household items. For example, plastic bottles filled with water are good substitutes for dumbbells. You can use them to exercise your arms and shoulders by doing biceps curls, shoulder shrugs, arm rows, or arm lifts.

Many highly effective muscle-strengthening exercises use the body's own weight as resistance. Pushups are a good example. You can do them standing up and pushing your body away from a wall. It is even more challenging to do the exercise against a desk or the back of a chair. Finally, if your arm strength permits it, you can do pushups with your hands on the floor. To strengthen your leg muscles, one of the best exercises is stair climbing. Other good leg exercises can be done by straightening and lifting your legs alternately while sitting on a chair, or by repeatedly getting up and sitting down on the edge of your chair. Stomach crunches are the best exercises for the stomach muscles. Lie on your back with your knees bent and your feet flat on the floor. Protect your neck by placing your hands lightly against the back of your neck, and curl up as far as you can, using only your stomach muscles. Remember not to strain your neck or shoulders.

Isometrics are another important subgroup of muscle-strengthening exercises. They involve tightening a particular muscle group and holding the position for a number of seconds. You can do isometrics by applying pressure against stationary objects or an opposing body part. Pushing against a doorjamb, pulling up on the chair you are sitting on, and pressing your palms against each other are examples of isometric exercises. Isometrics are very useful in that they can be performed almost any place without special equipment.

The Recommended Readings section of this book lists a

number of books and other references that will help you learn about different types of exercises in more detail. The implementation strategies in the next section of this chapter will help you incorporate physical activity into your daily life. They are simple techniques that you can start doing today.

Optimize Your Everyday Activities

It is extremely important that you increase your level of physical activity gradually. In this way, it will become a welcome and natural part of your life. You can begin by combining mild forms of exercise with everyday tasks. For example, park your car a little farther from your shopping destination, or take the stairs instead of the elevator. This will establish a connection between your normal activities and exercise. As you increase your level of physical activity, you will build more muscle, lose fat, and improve your fitness level. The benefits of fewer headaches and an improved sense of well-being will reinforce your efforts. Eventually, you will regard your headaches as something from the dark past, rather than as something to fear and anticipate.

If you currently enjoy some form of physical activity, you are already ahead of the game. Just be sure to maintain a level that will last your entire lifetime. Some of you may not be at the stage where you look forward to jogging, skiing, or working out, but if you follow some of the strategies discussed in this chapter, you will improve your level of physical activity. And—believe it or not—you will develop a taste for exercise.

STAYING ON TRACK

You know that in order to prevent headaches, you must increase your physical activity and improve your level of physical fitness. But until your new program becomes a natural part of your everyday routine, you may need some help staying on track. The following sections discuss some time-tested strategies to help you implement and maintain a more active lifestyle.

Begin Slowly

No one changes from a couch potato to an athlete overnight. In fact, to ensure a successful transition to a more active life, it is essential that you proceed slowly at the beginning. Fortunately, even if your sedentary habits are long established, it is never too late to start enjoying a healthy and active life, free of headaches. Be aware that you will probably go through various stages before you begin a regular program of exercise. At first, you may scoff at any suggestion that you increase your physical activity. But weight gain, various ailments, or the greater wisdom that sometimes comes with age will bring you to the stage of contemplation. This is when many people give up because they think that it is too late or not worth the effort. However, you now know that it is never too late. Once you reach the stage where you are ready to do something, you may have to apply various strategies to prevent a return to your sedentary habits. Just keep reminding yourself that by taking small incremental steps, you can achieve any lifestyle modification you desire.

Keep an Exercise Journal

It is a good idea to keep an exercise journal because it will help you track your progress, which keeps things in perspective. If you summarize the results of your exercise program at the end of each month and compare them with previous months, you will be pleasantly surprised to see how much you have increased your level of physical activity. Pay attention to any improvements in your physical fitness, decrease in body fat, weight loss, and improvements in your resting heart rate and general well-being.

Find an Exercise Buddy

The saying, "A shared pleasure is a doubled pleasure, a shared burden is half a burden," certainly applies to physical activity. Try to find a friend, an exercise buddy, who is also motivated to exercise. This has two major benefits. First, being able to talk to someone while walking, biking, or gardening can make it more fun. When the activity gets more challenging, having someone around to share the burden is a great help. In addition, having a partner usually creates a "moral" commitment to the activity for both participants. It is much easier to find an excuse to skip a day than it is to tell your partner that you can't make it. In addition to disappointing a friend, you may also lose face—a situation most of us try to avoid.

Keep Exercise Interesting

Activities that have some competitive aspect to them—that is, playing some form of game against an opponent or measuring improvements in your performance—are much easier to sustain over long periods of time than regimented workout sessions. But workouts can supplement your everyday physical activities, and there are ways to make them more interesting. A great way to take the boredom out of exercise is to combine it with music. A lively beat usually entices people to start moving. Dancing to music is one of the oldest forms of enjoyment, and you can do it in many different settings and at any age. You may want to consider buying an exercise videocassette. There are many such products on the market, each providing a unique style and approach to get you started. This provides for a more structured environment, demonstrates different types of exercises, and conveys a sense of excitement and joy derived from physical activity.

Make a Schedule

In order to get the full benefit of physical activities, you should do them on a regular basis. A spontaneous decision to go for a bike ride or a game of golf is fine, but it is no substitute for some form of regular activity. What you choose to do is entirely up to you, but you must decide when you will do it. Many activities will schedule themselves more or less automatically. If you are mowing your lawn on a weekly basis, the overgrown yard will remind you to do it. If you are used to walking your dog each morning or evening, she will make sure you don't forget. But many activities do not have a natural schedule. If you tell someone that it would be great to get together the following week for a game of squash or a bike ride, it will probably never happen. If you make up your mind to walk three times a week, pick the three days, decide on the time, and put them on your calendar. Do the same for any activity you want to add to your daily or weekly routine.

CONCLUSION

An adequate level of daily physical activity is essential to headache prevention. Making exercise fun is the key to making it an indispensable part of your life. Now that you have learned how to develop a taste for increased physical activity, you are ready to explore the impact of stress on the chemistry of the body and the importance of reducing chronic stress. Exercise is also very helpful for stress reduction because it eases many of the harmful effects of stress. The next chapter will help you begin phase three of my program.

CHAPTER 5

Chronic Stress and Headache

*There is nothing either good or bad,
but thinking makes it so.*

—William Shakespeare

Occasional stress is not harmful to health. In fact, the stress response is a survival mechanism that prepares the body to deal with an impending threat or other pressure. When we are faced with a threatening situation, our bodies go into a state called the *fight-or-flight response*, which mobilizes all our energy and resources for an immediate fight or escape. On the other hand, a constant barrage of stress, or *chronic* stress, causes many problems, and one of the most common is headache. This chapter will teach you how to manage chronic stress so that it becomes a motivating force, rather than a source of headaches. Before presenting the basic approach and strategies for stress management, I will explore the impact of stress the body's chemistry.

STRESS AND BODY CHEMISTRY

Stress is a stimulus or pressure that can interfere with the body's equilibrium, or homeostasis. In the health sciences, we call these pressures and stimuli *stressors*. And stress, or more precisely, the *stress response*, refers to the body's reaction to stressors. An encounter with a vicious dog and an impending deadline at work are two examples of stressors. The heart pounding, sweating, and muscle tenseness are normal stress reactions of the body.

Occasional Stress

The brain constantly monitors and adjusts the internal processes of the body. As it does this, it sends messages to various organs of the body through the *nervous system* and through the release of hormones. Nerves transmit signals within fractions of a second. Thus, when the brain detects an immediate danger, it makes the heart race almost instantaneously. It takes considerably more time to release hormones from a gland, transport them through the bloodstream, and wait for them to be detected. However, hormones can remain in the bloodstream and continue functioning for many hours after they have been released.

We are all familiar with the immediate reactions to stress. The heart starts beating faster as the blood vessels narrow, which increases blood pressure and supplies more oxygen and nutrients to the muscles. At the same time, breathing becomes faster as the body attempts to replenish oxygen in the blood. All skeletal muscles, especially those of the neck and shoulders, become tense and ready for action, and perspiration increases to cool the body. The pupils dilate to improve vision, and digestion and other nonvital processes stop to preserve energy.

While this is going on, the brain releases several hormones—in particular, adrenaline and *noradrenaline*—that intensify the reactions produced by the nervous system. These include increasing heart rate, blood pressure, perspiration, body temperature, blood clotting, and levels of blood sugar and blood fat. The body's response to stressful stimuli occurs within seconds. Once the situation returns to normal, the stress signals are no longer sent to the brain, and the body slowly returns to its previous state. This is a perfectly normal and natural reaction and is not damaging to the body.

Chronic Stress

When stressful events occur frequently, or when they are of long duration and extreme intensity, stress becomes chronic. Constant stress can lead to biochemical imbalances and potentially serious health problems. Why? The body needs time to recover from a stress response. It must clear the various stress-related hormones from the bloodstream and permit all the biochemical processes and organs to return to a normal state. When stress is ongoing, the body remains in a permanent state of high alert; and this can lead to depression, anxiety, insomnia, and a number of other problems.

From the headache perspective, the most important biochemical changes caused by chronic stress are increased levels of blood fat and increased blood clotting. This is the result of hormones such as adrenaline, noradrenaline, and cortisol, which are released into the bloodstream when you are under stress. Increased levels of blood fat and increased platelet clustering cause a lowering of serotonin levels, which results in vasodilatation and headaches. Another important factor known to cause or exacerbate headaches is increased tension of neck and shoulder muscles, which is part of the natural stress response.

But headaches are not only the result of chronic stress; they can also cause chronic stress. How? The fear of future pain causes biochemical imbalances in the body—that is, a stress response. This, in turn, increases the risk of headaches and results in an ongoing cycle of stress and headaches. To prevent headaches and other chronic health problems, your long-term goal must be to keep your stress level within the optimum range. This means that you must reduce all your controllable stressors to a minimum, especially stressors that might be *imaginary*. What is an imaginary stressor? It is any stressor that is a product of your thoughts—for example, worrying about losing your job or agonizing about events that may never happen.

WHY OUR LIVES ARE STRESSFUL

All higher level organisms experience stress. As I have said, stress protects us from danger and helps us adapt to the environment. Why is it that humans manage to turn stress into something that is harmful? A major part of the answer lies in our intelligence, which permits us to imagine threats and demands that may never occur. A dog will have a stress reaction when faced with a snake, and so will most humans. However, people can also visualize an encounter with a snake and experience the same stress reaction to the imaginary snake as though it were real. Worse yet, only humans can imagine all the consequences of such an encounter—the pain of the bite, their impending death, and the consequences for their families.

Our intelligence also makes a major difference in how we deal with stress. Animals in the wild always follow their instincts. If they perceive something as dangerous or uncomfortable, they run away or try to avoid it. But we humans have learned to suppress many of our natural instincts. When faced with a tight deadline or an intimidating boss, we do not simply run away, because our ability to foresee the consequences prevents us from doing what our body is prepared to do—namely, fight or run away. Instead, we force ourselves to overcome our aversions and suppress any immediate need to relieve stress.

In order to combat chronic stress, we must attempt to decrease the number and intensity of our stressors. One way to do this is to control our thought processes. This will avoid unnecessary muscle tension, and it will keep blood fat levels low.

While some stress is the result of circumstances beyond our control, such as illness, death of a loved one, or acts of violence, much stress is self-imposed. For example, we often make unreasonable commitments in our social and professional lives. The common root of most stressors in our society is time—or rather, the lack of it.

Why is there such a chronic shortage of time? One reason may be that we invest our time poorly. For example, some of us invest a great deal of our time in making money. Why? Technology constantly bombards us with new products, and advertising tries to make us feel that we should have all of them. So, we need more money and we invest more and more time in its endless pursuit. Furthermore, the pursuit of money is often interconnected with the quest for fame and power; and all of these are major sources of stress.

There is nothing wrong with wishing to be successful and respected. After all, this is often the driving force behind human progress. But it is a good idea to question whether it is worth the cost. After all, what are the important things in life? Time spent with our families and friends, hobbies, entertainment, and good health. To quote Mahatma Gandhi, "There is more to life than increasing its speed."

The key to deciding how to invest your time and thus control your stress is to find the right balance between long-term and short-term goals. We all need goals in life, but people often over-commit themselves when they accept too many short-term challenges that they are unable to meet. Instead, it is better to see life as a continuing series of steps, each representing a goal. Reaching each intermediate goal fills you with satisfaction and provides the necessary motivation to keep going.

TYPES OF STRESS-MANAGEMENT TECHNIQUES

Despite the barrage of stressors in our lives, there are many ways to reduce stress. Physical exercise is an excellent stress reducer because it uses up the excess blood fat and blood sugar that the brain has released into the bloodstream to prepare the body for a fight-or-flight situation. But there are also a number of other highly effective stress-reduction techniques, which we will explore in the following sections.

Relaxation Techniques

Relaxation techniques involve mental and breathing exercises that offer immediate and long-term relief from stress. These active relaxation techniques work by calming your body and mind as they disconnect from all thought processes. Listening to music—not just as background noise while doing something else, but in a concentrated manner—is a good first step. Similarly, trying to appreciate nature by actively absorbing and admiring its minute details is also extremely relaxing. The following sections describe some techniques that are simple to do and can be done any time you feel stressed.

Deep Breathing

Deep breathing is a highly effective form of active relaxation that produces the fastest results. It is also called *abdominal breathing,* because the breathing process involves the abdomen rather than the chest. The main purpose of deep breathing is to increase the supply of oxygen to the lungs and thus prevent an increase in heart rate and muscle tension. The first step is to learn a simple breathing routine that lasts just a few seconds. You can find examples in most books on relaxation or stress management, or you can develop your own technique. For example, close your eyes and take a slow, deep breath using mostly your abdomen. Hold your breath for two or three seconds, and as you slowly exhale, imagine something pleasant. Repeat this three times.

Once you know your routine, you should incorporate it into your daily life so that you do not have to think about doing it. The best way to do this is to associate it with another activity, such as entering your workplace, going into a meeting, taking a break, or stopping at a red light, so that it is triggered automatically. Once it becomes a habit, make it more elaborate and more frequent—you can design your own routines to fit your schedule.

The main advantage of deep breathing as a relaxation technique is that you can practice it anywhere and anytime, without preparation, and without special equipment. And it is easy to do. Deep breathing is extremely versatile—you can do it for a few seconds to prepare for a difficult telephone call, presentation, or confrontation; or you can do it for longer periods of time to wind down after work or to relax before going to sleep. The most important thing is to make it as automatic as regular breathing.

Progressive Muscle Relaxation

Progressive muscle relaxation trains you to recognize the difference between tense muscles and relaxed muscles, which helps you relax all your skeletal muscle groups. You generally start by consciously tensing and releasing the muscles in your hands and arms, and then continue the process with the muscles of your head, shoulders, chest, and so on until you have relaxed your entire body. Each session of progressive muscle relaxation generally takes a few minutes. By concentrating on tensing and relaxing your muscles, you will naturally disconnect from stress-producing thoughts. This is a very useful technique to use before falling asleep.

Autogenics

Autogenics trains your body and mind to respond to verbal relaxation commands, which you issue to yourself. You perform each session in a relaxed position, sitting or lying down, with your eyes closed. Through a steady stream of verbal commands that you silently repeat to yourself, you can produce certain feelings, such as heaviness or warmth in your arms, legs, or stomach. You can also calm your breathing and your heart rate.

Visualization

Many people combine autogenics with visualization techniques. One common form of visualization is to concentrate on the image of a pleasant surrounding, such as a beach, and think about the sounds, smells, or sights associated with that place. This helps you detach your thoughts from reality and relax your mind. You can use visualization very effectively to control fear or anxiety. Let's say you are on a flight that is experiencing an unpleasant level of turbulence. In such a situation, you would visualize yourself at the end of the flight, stepping off the plane to begin your vacation, greeting your friends and relatives, or whatever pleasant expectations you might have.

Biofeedback

Biofeedback is an extremely effective technique for treating headaches. The technique lets you monitor certain changes in your body, such as body temperature, brain-wave activity, and heartbeat. This is done using devices such as skin electrodes or a thermometer. Normally, the brain automatically controls physiological changes; but through biofeedback, you can learn to induce and control such changes at will.

Meditation

Meditation, like autogenics, is also performed in a relaxed position with your eyes closed. Your aim is to focus your attention on one thing, such as an object, a sound, or your breathing, which enables you to relax by emptying your mind of all other thoughts. Meditation is a highly effective relaxation technique, but it requires some practice to master.

Self-Hypnosis

Self-hypnosis is an advanced relaxation technique that enables you to enter a state of deep relaxation as you respond to your own verbal suggestions or commands. Its main purpose is to let you experience your thoughts and images as if they were real, causing the same physiological reactions as the actual situation. How can this help? The self-induced relaxation counters your stress response. You can bring many beneficial changes to your body's biochemistry by imagining positive situations and letting your body experience them as if they were real.

Coping Skills

Another way to reduce stress is to learn new ways of coping with stressors. First, however, you must be able to recognize and analyze your stress symptoms. This can be as simple as going over the day's experiences to identify any stress-producing situations as well as your physiological, psychological, and behavioral symptoms. These may include headache, fatigue, depression, anxiety, or irritability. You can then apply other techniques such as *rational thinking* to decide whether your worries were based on objective reality or something that has a very low probability of occurring.

Once you better understand your stressors, you can start taking steps toward reducing stress. One way to do this is through *positive self-talk.* As the term suggests, you provide yourself a boost of confidence by praising and encouraging your own actions. It has been shown that you can greatly influence the outcome of many situations by telling yourself what you wish to happen and by convincing yourself that it will happen. Remember that the way you respond to most situations is entirely up to you. Thomas Edison gives us an excellent example of positive self-talk: "I have not failed 10,000 times; I have successfully found 10,000 ways that will not work."

Other examples of coping skills include learning to *refute irrational ideas* by replacing them with realistic statements, and *thought stopping,* which involves concentrating on an unwanted thought and then suddenly stopping and emptying your mind. You then substitute a pleasant thought for the unwanted one.

Assertiveness Training

Assertiveness training includes a set of life skills aimed at strengthening those aspects of your personality that make you vulnerable or ineffective in interacting with others. For example, some people must learn to disagree with others when it is appropriate to do so; others may have to learn to say "no" to too many demands. And others may have to learn how to ask for emotional support. Such coping skills help people get their personal or professional life under control and reduce stress. Assertiveness training is available through courses or seminars, and there are many excellent books for self-study.

Life-Management Skills

Life-management skills are simple yet very effective stress-reducers. They involve deciding on priorities, planning activities, and learning how to become more organized. Specific skills may include goal-setting and -planning, time- and money-management, and problem-solving.

Another type of life-management training aims at improving your *communication skills*. These include your body language, which carries important messages about your feelings and attitudes; your listening skills; and your ability to express yourself concisely, clearly, and assertively in a way that is not threatening, sarcastic, or condescending.

GUIDELINES FOR MANAGING STRESS

There are two main groups of relaxation techniques, which are included in the Stress-Management Technique Pyramid in Figure 5.1 on page 99. The first group includes simple techniques that you can perform with no or minimal training, such as deep breathing or progressive muscle relaxation. You should be able to start applying these today and continue them indefinitely to prevent or manage stress. The more advanced relaxation techniques require some degree of training and practice.

Life skills are also divided into two groups. Everyday life skills include many simple techniques that you can apply immediately. Specialized life skills include more systematic programs in assertiveness training, coping skills,

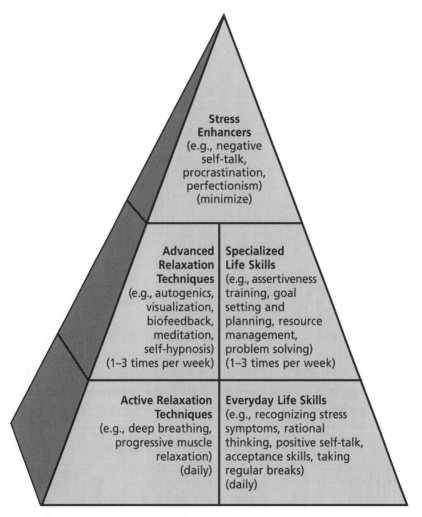

Figure 5.1. The Stress-Management Technique Pyramid

and life-management skills. Many people have these skills naturally, but others may benefit from formal instruction or training.

The tip of the Stress-Management Technique Pyramid represents activities that promote or enhance stress. Obviously, you must keep these activities to a minimum. Typical examples include procrastination, perfectionism, doing too many things at the same time, or negative self-talk.

You will find several books on stress management in the Recommended Readings at the back of this book. They offer hundreds of simple tips on preventing and coping with stress plus a wide range of techniques, from simple breathing exercises to a complete restructuring of your psyche. The implementation strategies in the following section will then help you incorporate the various stress-prevention and coping skills into your daily routine.

Categorizing Your Level of Stress

The level of stress in your life is equal to the gap between the *demands* imposed on you and the financial, physical, emotional, or psychological *resources* available to meet those demands. The stress-elimination choices we make should narrow that gap.

It is useful to realize that there are several levels of stress. The lowest level is *optimum* stress. This type of stress is necessary for continuous adaptation to the environment and as a motivational force for optimum performance.

The next level is called *manageable* stress, implying that the stress level is not optimum, but can still be held in check with proper stress-management techniques. Manageable stress may result from a new job, a marriage, the birth of a child, the purchase of a new home, or any number of normal life events involving a major change.

Adjusting to a new situation often requires some time, and during this time, you may experience *excessive* stress. This causes significant wear and tear on your body and mind. But as long as the rise in demands or the drop in resources is not too sharp, you will be able to narrow the gap and regain a steady state of optimum stress.

The most serious situation occurs when the gap between the demands and the resources is too wide and you cannot immediately repair it. Excessive stress leads to a state of *burnout,* where depression, anxiety, and other emotional as well as physiological health problems make daily living extremely difficult. The goal of successful stress management is to keep the gap between demands and resources within optimum range. The following sections offer some ideas so you can achieve that goal.

Identify Your Stressors

One way to deal with your stressors is to group them into *controllable stressors* and *uncontrollable stressors.* As the name implies, controllable stressors are those that you are able to avoid or eliminate. Examples of such stressors are your choice of friends or your attempts to keep up with your neighbors. If these are sources of irritation, the best approach is to avoid them. Examples of uncontrollable stressors are serious illness, death in the family, or divorce. But under certain circumstances, even mundane problems can be stressors. In cases such as these, the only reasonable approach is to apply stress-reduction techniques to change your perception of the situation.

Integrate Stress Management With Other Activities

Given the busy schedule that most people have, it can be a challenge to find the time to practice active relaxation techniques or to learn new stress-management skills. The key is to integrate stress management with your daily activities so that it causes minimal disruptions to your life. Similar to developing a taste for healthier nutrition and more physical activity, this must be done gradually so that stress management becomes an unobtrusive and automatic part of your daily routine.

Just as physical work requires frequent breaks to relax your body, mental activity requires frequent breaks to relax your mind. Remember that the body is more likely to demand that you take a break, because at some point, you feel physically tired and your muscles refuse to cooperate until they have a chance to regain their energy. Your brain is more forgiving. It will allow you to sit at your desk or in front of a computer screen for many hours without a break. In fact, the more intellectually challenging the task you are working on, the less likely you are to take a break. But there is no doubt that efficiency decreases with time. By taking frequent breaks, you refresh your mind, perhaps gain a new perspective on the problem at hand, and are likely to finish your task faster than by running a mental marathon.

The main problem is that many tasks simply do not lend themselves to interruptions. There is always one more sentence to write or one more experiment to try, and it seems that a break would disturb the train of thought. The best way to remember to take a break is to use some form of alarm that will remind you that another hour has passed by. If you are afraid of losing your train of thought, just make a note of where you are so you do not have to backtrack when you return from your break. Do not ignore the alarm. Interrupt your work promptly, if only for a minute, and do some stretching as well as some form of relaxation exercise—simple deep breathing will do. This will make you much more productive in the end.

In addition, if you are financially able to take a day off from work every week and a few brief vacations each year, you would go a long way toward eliminating chronic stress. When you are not at work, you should not worry about an unfinished project or think about what you must do the following day. That is not rest. Whenever the thought of work pops into your mind, try to drive it away. Train yourself to refuse to consider anything related to work during your free time.

STAYING ON TRACK

We have all made up our minds to implement changes in our lives, but we often have trouble sticking with it. However, when it comes to reducing stress, it is essential that you stay on track. It's the only way to eliminate your headaches once and for all. The following sections offer some strategies that will help you make the necessary adjustments so that you can enjoy a less stressful life.

Begin Slowly

Unlike changing your diet or increasing physical activity, which must be done gradually to prevent discomfort or harm to your body, a sudden stress-relaxation regime will not cause any physical problems. Nevertheless, for psychological reasons, you should introduce relaxation techniques gradually. Attempting an advanced technique without having explored simple breathing is bound to lead to disappointment and failure. Even if it starts out as exciting, the novelty will soon wear off and the difficulties of mastering any advanced technique will force you to give up.

If you are already applying some relaxation technique, continue on your path by further expanding your mental resources. If you are new to this domain, then follow some of the strategies in this chapter to make stress reduction part of your daily routine. But always remember that you should start with something simple such as deep breathing. As time goes on, you can introduce muscle relaxation exercises or autogenics. At the same time, you can start working on some very simple life skills to help you solve recurring problems at home or at work. Each person is different and there is no universal recipe for stress management. You must discover for yourself which activities work. However, keep in mind that the most important aspect of successful stress management is to begin slowly and to develop the habit of daily stress-reduction exercises.

Make a Schedule

Some stress-management techniques are designed to deal with stress that is already present. For example, you can use relaxation and concentration techniques whenever you feel tense. But remember that to achieve the greatest stress reduction, you must engage in stress-prevention activities on a regular basis.

When you set up your schedule, select specific days and times for your relaxation exercises and put them on your calendar just as you would a weekly meeting. You can also combine relaxation with other regularly scheduled activities. This will help you train yourself to do them automatically and unobtrusively. To begin, pick three to five daily events, and do a very simple breathing exercise before or after each. If you have difficulty falling asleep, learn how to do some simple muscle-relaxation or autogenic exercises, and practice these when you are ready to go to sleep. You will be amazed at how well they work and how much better you will feel in the morning.

Write It Down

The human mind works sequentially in that it can only work on one thought at a time. If your brain must process several things at once, it must switch back and forth between them. Such a mental juggling act can be very stressful. However, a pen and a piece of paper can go a long way to alleviate this problem. Have these handy at all times. As you are going through a thinking process and some unrelated problem pops into your head, quickly jot it down, and then return to the problem at hand.

A pen and paper are also very useful for writing down certain positive things that happen during the day. Time tends to distort reality—what may have seemed of great significance a month ago may be of absolutely no consequence today, or vice versa. Writing things down helps you keep things in perspective. If you feel angry or depressed, it will be difficult to recall any positive aspects of your past few days or weeks. Writing down any praise or compliment you receive and all the successes and accomplishments that you achieve on a daily basis will help you recall these when you are in distress. You can use them as part of your positive self-talk to improve your state of mind.

Talk to Someone

Anger, fear, and sadness are all emotions that cause a lot of stress. Each manifests itself differently, but each can keep growing on its own, even after the initial stimulus has disappeared. The best way to make sure that you stay on track and keep stress at a minimum is to talk to someone—a friend, a relative, or a professional. A second opinion can help change your outlook in ways that you could not have imagined yourself.

Sometimes, it is helpful to talk to the person who is the subject of your worries, anger, or fear. This is very difficult, but once you have broken the initial barrier, the situation may quickly change for the better as you begin to see things from the other person's perspective. And this can go a long way toward relieving a stressful situation.

Confront Your Fears and Anxieties

Fear comes from many sources. Some fears may be a reaction to a threat of physical harm, and others may be strictly psychological or emotional fears. But whatever its source, fear is a stressor. One of the best ways to overcome psychological fears is to expose yourself to the source of your perceived danger, starting at a very low dose. Of course, this will cause short-term stress, but as you gradually increase your exposure, you become more confident and your level of chronic stress will diminish. For example, if you are uncomfortable or anxious about speaking in front of others, you can gradually increase your level of confidence through repeated exposure and practice. Start with a small audience, perhaps a few friends or family members, and talk about a subject with which you are entirely comfortable. After a few repetitions, you will start feeling confident and can work your way up to more challenging presentations. With time, you will become desensitized and gain the necessary confidence to realize that you can overcome your fears.

CONCLUSION

By now, you have learned a great deal about the effects of stress on your body and how it can cause headaches. In addition, you have an assortment of guidelines and strategies to help you incorporate stress-management techniques into your everyday life. The following chapter will show you how you can monitor the effectiveness of your lifestyle changes.

CHAPTER 6

Measures of Success

If you only add a little at a time, it will soon become a big heap.

—Hesiod

Throughout the previous chapters, you have been urged to adapt slowly to any changes in your nutrition, physical activity, and stress-management techniques. Unfortunately, time has a way of blurring your memory, and this makes it difficult to track any progress you make, especially when the progress is gradual. For example, if you had to recall now how many headaches you experienced last month, your estimate may be accurate. In a few months, perhaps your headaches will have decreased significantly, and you may be hard-pressed to guess how much you have really improved. Nonetheless, you can fortify your long-term memory by keeping written records of your progress.

MONITORING HEADACHES

The primary goal of this book is to help you decrease the number and severity of your headaches. For this reason, you should keep a written record of your headaches and use of headache medication. An easy way to do this is to keep a simple headache journal. Make several copies of The Headache Journal in Figure 6.1 on page 109—one for each month. Make an entry before going to bed. If you forget one day, try to recall it in the morning; but the longer you skip, the less reliable your recollection will be.

If you did not have a headache, simply leave the line blank. If you did have a headache, place a check mark in the first column. In the second column, enter the *intensity* of the headache. You can rate headache intensity using a scale from one to three, where the different numbers have the following meaning:

1. Slight headache, can be ignored.

2. Moderate headache, resulting in noticeable discomfort.

3. Severe headache, interfering with work or daily activity.

These codes are only suggestions. You can decide on the exact meaning of each value based on the type and the perception of your headache. You can even devise your own scale, perhaps increasing the number of possible values to have a finer resolution. It is important that you write down your definitions and use them consistently over time to track any changes.

The third column in the headache journal records the *duration* of the headache, which you should record in terms of hours. This may be difficult to do, but even approximate values will be useful. In case you experience more than one headache during the day, simply add the hours together. But if you experience frequent headaches, you can devise your own way of keeping track of them.

The fourth column records the amount of headache medication you have taken that day. If you only take one type, then simply enter the number of tablets or capsules. If you use more than one medication, you may want to split the medication column so that there is one for each type.

Day	Headache (check mark)	Intensity (0–3)	Duration (hours)	Medication (dose)
Month:				
1				
2				
3				
4				
5				
6				
7				
8				
9				
10				
11				
12				
13				
14				
15				
16				
17				
18				
19				
20				
21				
22				
23				
24				
25				
26				
27				
28				
29				
30				
31				
Sum				
Average:				

Figure 6.1. The Headache Journal

At the end of each month, add the values in each column, and enter the results in the appropriate space at the bottom of the journal. The sum in the first column represents the number of days you have had headaches during the month. For the second and third columns, you can compute the *average* intensity and duration of your headaches for the month. The sum in the fourth column gives the total amount of headache medication you have taken that month. Keeping a headache journal means additional work, but you do not have to keep it indefinitely. It is important only during the first few months while you are in the process of modifying your lifestyle. Once you have established new habits and have settled in a new routine, your headaches will have greatly diminished or disappeared completely, and you can discontinue your headache journal. I recommend keeping the journal for a period of three to six months.

MONITORING OTHER CHANGES

Your main goal is to eliminate headaches, but it will take several weeks before you notice any significant improvement. This can be discouraging. But you must remember that many changes will take place in your body as soon as you start adapting to a healthier lifestyle. Monitoring these changes during the first few months will provide you with feedback and will tell you whether you are on the right track. This will also give you the necessary encouragement to continue your new approach.

Monitoring Body Fat

Some people find it helpful to monitor their body fat as well as the incidence of headaches, because high blood fat is a major cause of headaches. As you decrease the amount of fat you eat and increase your physical activity, the composition of your body will start to change. In particular, you will build up more muscle mass, which will replace stored fat in your body. In short, you will have decreased your percentage of body fat.

The actual percentage of fat in your body is the best indicator of dietary fat intake, exercise habits, and stress perception. A healthy male body should be 8 to 15 percent fat, and a healthy female body should be 13 to 23 percent fat.

The easiest way to determine your percentage of body fat is to use a weight scale with a built-in body-fat analyzer. A number of simple and relatively inexpensive models—around one hundred dollars—are on the market. Another simple, effective way to measure body fat is to determine your waist-to-hips ratio. You can do this by measuring the circumference of your waist and your hips and then divide the first value by the second. The ratio should be below 0.75 for women and below 0.85 for men. Anything above this indicates increased risk of chronic disease, including headache.

Monitoring Digestive Problems

The most common ailments resulting from an unhealthy lifestyle affect digestion—for example, heartburn, constipation, diarrhea, and flatulence. As you are adapting your lifestyle to one that includes more balanced nutrition, increased physical activity, and less stress, you will experience fewer digestive problems. Monitoring these changes serves as an important indicator that changes are occurring. Remember that if you modify your diet too suddenly, you may experience a temporary increase in certain digestive problems. But with time, you will be pleasantly surprised to see your digestive problems diminish or completely disappear.

Monitoring Psychological Symptoms

With stress management and increased physical activity, many psychological problems such as fatigue, anxiety, depression, or insomnia should start to resolve themselves.

It can be helpful to keep track of these improvements by keeping a journal.

Monitoring Cardiovascular System Changes

The suggested lifestyle changes will have immediate beneficial effects on your cardiovascular system. You can easily monitor changes in your blood pressure and resting heart rate. To determine your blood pressure at home, you need a blood pressure monitor, which is available in most pharmacies. Each measurement yields two numbers, one called the *systolic* pressure and the other called *diastolic*. Normal blood pressure in the average healthy adult is about 120/80—pronounced 120 over 80. This means that the systolic pressure is 120 and the diastolic pressure is 80.

Your resting heart rate is easily determined without any special equipment. Simply find your pulse by feeling the wrist of one hand with the fingertips of the other hand. Then count the number of heartbeats per minute. A healthy heart rate will be between 50 and 65 beats per minute, depending on your age and gender. When taking your blood pressure or heart rate, you should be in a resting position and should not have been doing any physical activity for some time before the measurement. The best time to take them is in the morning or after a long resting period.

CONCLUSION

Monitoring your progress is an important part of a successful headache-prevention program. Observing gradual changes taking place will reassure you that your new lifestyle is working for you, and it will give you the encouragement to continue. You will find that you will have fewer, less severe headaches.

Conclusion

The information in this book has given you an opportunity to think about your present lifestyle and improve it as much as possible so that you can eliminate headaches from your life. The key to good health is to take responsibility for your own health. You know your body better than anyone else does. Learn to recognize the biochemical changes that manifest themselves as headaches, and take steps to get them back into balance.

This is possible only if you take a positive approach. Changing your diet, increasing physical activity, and reducing your stress are your main long-term goals. But as long as you see them as restrictions or impositions on your present life, you will not be able to sustain the changes for very long. The various strategies presented in this book will help you develop gradual changes in your taste for a different healthier lifestyle. It may take months, but they will not be months of deprivation or resistance to activities you dislike. Instead, your life will proceed with a minimum of disruption and discomfort. And in the end, you will emerge with a much healthier body and a positive outlook for a bright future, free of headaches.

APPENDIX A

Recommended Sources of Nutrients

The following tables list the sources of some of the most important nutrients in terms of headache prevention. The foods listed are not necessarily those with the highest amounts of specific nutrients, because some high-nutrient foods may contain less desirable components. Thus, the foods we recommend in these tables are the best for overall well-balanced nutrition, and they are the most beneficial for headache prevention. Since one of your main nutritional goals is to limit your intake of fat, the tables also list the caloric and fat content of each food.

MAGNESIUM				
Food	Serving Size	Magnesium	Calories	Fat
Rye flour (dark)	1 cup	317 mg	415	3.4 g
Artichoke (boiled)	one (medium)	180 mg	150	0.5 g
Pumpkin/squash seeds (dried)	1 oz	152 mg	153	13.0 g
Soybeans (boiled)	1 cup	148 mg	298	15.4 g
Tofu (soybean curd)	½ cup	128 mg	94	5.9 g
Brown rice (cooked)	1 cup	86 mg	218	1.6 g
Kidney beans (boiled)	1 cup	80 mg	225	0.9 g

Food	Serving Size	Magnesium	Calories	Fat
Spinach (boiled)	½ cup	78 mg	21	0.2 g
Banana	one (medium)	33 mg	105	0.5 g
Whole-wheat bread	one slice	24 mg	69	1.2 g

VITAMIN C

Food	Serving Size	Vitamin C	Calories	Fat
Bell pepper (yellow)	one (large)	341 mg	50	0.4 g
Papaya	one (medium)	188 mg	119	0.4 g
Black currant	½ cup	101 mg	35	0.2 g
Grapefruit (pink or red)	one (medium)	84 mg	78	0.2 g
Orange (navel)	one (medium)	75 mg	60	0.1 g
Kiwifruit	one (medium)	74 mg	46	0.3 g
Broccoli (boiled)	½ cup	58 mg	22	0.3 g
Brussels sprouts (boiled)	½ cup	48 mg	30	0.4 g
Strawberries	1 cup	84 mg	45	0.6 g
Cantaloupe (pieces)	1 cup	68 mg	56	0.4 g

VITAMIN A

Food	Serving Size	Vitamin A	Calories	Fat
Sweet potato (boiled)	½ cup	2,796 RE*	172	0.5 g
Pumpkin (canned)	½ cup	2,691 RE	41	0.3 g
Carrots (boiled)	½ cup	1,915 RE	35	0.1 g
Mango	one (medium)	805 RE	135	0.6 g
Spinach (boiled)	½ cup	737 RE	21	0.2 g
Cantaloupe (pieces)	1 cup	515 RE	56	0.4 g
Beet greens (boiled)	½ cup	367 RE	19	0.1 g

Food	Serving Size	Vitamin A	Calories	Fat
Persimmon	one (medium)	365 RE	118	0.3 g
Apricots	three (medium)	277 RE	51	0.4 g
Prunes	ten (medium)	167 RE	201	0.4 g

*RE = micrograms of retinol equivalents

VITAMIN B₆ (PYRIDOXINE)

Food	Serving Size	Vitamin B₆	Calories	Fat
Rice bran	1 oz	1.15 mg	90	5.9 g
Chickpeas (garbanzos, canned)	1 cup	1.14 mg	286	2.7 g
Bran cereals	½ cup	0.90 mg	75	1.4 g
Avocado (Florida)	one (medium)	0.85 mg	340	27.0 g
Oatmeal (cooked)	one packet	0.74 mg	104	1.8 g
Potatoes (baked with skin)	one (medium)	0.70 mg	220	0.2 g
Banana	one (medium)	0.66 mg	105	0.5 g
Corn flakes	1 cup	0.50 mg	120	0.5 g
Figs (dried)	ten	0.42 mg	477	2.2 g
Sweet potato (boiled)	½ cup	0.40 mg	172	0.5 g

VITAMIN B₃ (NIACIN)

Food	Serving Size	Vitamin B₃	Calories	Fat
Tuna (canned in water)	3 oz	11.3 mg	99	0.7 g
Brewer's yeast	1 oz	10.7 mg	80	0.3 g
Bran cereals	½ cup	8.9 mg	75	1.4 g
Buckwheat flour	1 cup	7.4 mg	402	3.7 g
Halibut (broiled)	3 oz	6.1 mg	119	2.5 g

Food	Serving Size	Vitamin B₃	Calories	Fat
Corn flakes	1 cup	5.0 mg	120	0.5 g
Peanut butter (crunchy)	2 Tbsp	4.4 mg	188	16.0 g
Mushrooms (boiled)	½ cup	3.5 mg	21	0.4 g
Rice (medium grain, cooked)	1 cup	3.4 mg	242	0.4 g
Potatoes (baked with skin)	one (medium)	3.3 mg	220	0.2 g

VITAMIN B$_2$ (RIBOFLAVIN)				
Food	Serving Size	Vitamin B$_2$	Calories	Fat
Seaweed (spirulina, dried)	3.5 oz	3.67 mg	290	7.7g
Brewer's yeast	1 oz	1.21 mg	80	0.3 g
Bran cereals	½ cup	0.76 mg	75	1.4 g
Yogurt (nonfat)	1 cup	0.53 mg	127	0.4 g
Soybeans (boiled)	1 cup	0.49 mg	298	15.4 g
Corn flakes	1 cup	0.43 mg	120	0.5 g
Milk (nonfat)	1 cup	0.43 mg	90	0.6 g
Mushrooms (boiled)	½ cup	0.23 mg	21	0.4 g
Spinach (boiled)	½ cup	0.21 mg	21	0.2 g
Beet greens (boiled)	½ cup	0.21 mg	19	0.1 g

TRYPTOPHAN				
Food	Serving Size	Tryptophan	Calories	Fat
Seaweed (spirulina, dried)	3.5 oz	929 mg	290	7.7 g
Soybean nuts (dry roasted)	½ cup	494 mg	405	21.8 g

Food	Serving Size	Tryptophan	Calories	Fat
Cottage cheese (1% fat)	1 cup	312 mg	164	2.3 g
Whole-wheat flour	1 cup	254 mg	407	2.2 g
Navy beans (canned)	1 cup	233 mg	296	1.1 g
Buckwheat flour	1 cup	220 mg	402	3.7 g
Black beans (boiled)	1 cup	181 mg	227	0.9 g
Tofu (soybean curd)	½ cup	156 mg	94	5.9 g
Watermelon seeds (dried)	1 oz	111 mg	158	13.4 g
Almonds (dried)	1 oz	100 mg	165	14.6 g

DIETARY FIBER				
Food	Serving Size	Fiber	Calories	Fat
Rye flour (dark)	1 cup	28.9 g	415	3.4 g
Corn bran (raw)	⅓ cup	21.4 g	56	0.2 g
Figs (dried)	ten (medium)	17.4 g	477	2.2 g
Black beans (boiled)	1 cup	15.0 g	227	0.9 g
Pinto beans (boiled)	1 cup	14.7 g	234	0.9 g
Whole-wheat flour	1 cup	14.6 g	407	2.2 g
Refried beans (canned)	1 cup	13.4 g	238	3.2 g
Chickpeas (canned)	1 cup	10.6 g	286	2.7 g
Bran cereals	½ cup	8.3 g	75	1.4 g
Pear (with skin)	one (medium)	4.0 g	98	0.7 g

OMEGA-3 FATTY ACIDS				
Food	**Serving Size**	**Omega-3**	**Calories**	**Fat**
Flaxseed (linseed) oil	1 Tbsp	6.6 g	124	14.0 g
Walnuts	1 oz	1.9 g	172	16.0 g
Canola oil	1 Tbsp	1.6 g	124	14.0 g
Walnut oil	1 Tbsp	1.5 g	124	14.0 g
Soybeans (boiled)	1 cup	1.1 g	298	15.4 g
Salmon (broiled)	3 oz	2.0 g	175	10.5 g
Soybean oil	1 Tbsp	0.9 g	124	14.0 g
Tofu (soybean curd, firm)	½ cup	0.7 g	94	5.9 g
Soy milk	1 cup	0.4 g	79	4.6 g
Wheat germ	¼ cup	0.2 g	104	2.8 g

APPENDIX B

Recommended Readings

NUTRITION

Practical Guides and Cookbooks

Chelf, Vicki Rae and Dominique Biscotti. *The Sensuous Vegetarian Barbecue*. Garden City Park, NY: Avery Publishing Group, 1994.

Compestine, Ying Chang. *Secrets of Fat-Free Chinese Cooking*. Garden City Park, NY: Avery Publishing Group, 1999.

Horsley, Janet. *Bean Cuisine*. Garden City Park, NY: Avery Publishing Group, 1989.

Levin, James and Natalie Cederquist. *A Celebration of Wellness: A Cookbook for Vibrant Living*. Garden City Park, NY: Avery Publishing Group, 1995.

Messina, Mark, Virginia Messina, and Ken Setchel. *The Simple Soybean and Your Health*. Garden City Park, NY: Avery Publishing Group, 1994.

Paino, John and Lisa Messinger. *The Tofu Book*. Garden City Park, NY: Avery Publishing Group, 1991.

Rose, Gloria. *Low-fat Cooking for Good Health.* Garden City Park, NY: Avery Publishing Group, 1996.

Vegetarian Resource Group. *Vegetarian Journal's Guide to Natural Food Restaurants in the US and Canada.* Garden City Park, NY: Avery Publishing Group, 1998.

Woodruff, Sandra. *Secrets of Fat-Free Italian Cooking.* Garden City Park, NY: Avery Publishing Group, 1997.

Nutrtional Reference Books

Bellerson, Karen J. *The Complete and Up-to-Date Fat Book.* Garden City Park, NY: Avery Publishing Group, 1993.

Ulene, Art. *The Nutribase Nutrition Facts Desk Reference.* Garden City Park, NY: Avery Publishing Group, 1995.

Nutrition and Food Science

Krause, Mari V. and L. Kathleen Mohan. *Food, Nutrition, and Diet Therapy.* Philadelphia: W.B. Saunders Co., 1984.

Messina, Mark and Virginia Messina. *The Dietitian's Guide to Vegetarian Diets.* Gaithersburg, MD: Aspen Publishers, Inc., 1996.

Whitney, Eleanor N. and Sharon R. Rolfes. *Understanding Nutrition.* St. Paul, MN: West Publishing Co., 1993.

EXERCISE AND PHYSICAL ACTIVITY

Practical Guides and Fitness Programs

American College of Sports Medicine. *ACSM Fitness Book.* Champaign, IL: Human Kinetics, 1998.

Anderson, Bob. *Stretching.* Bolinas, CA: Sheller Publications, 1980.

Anderson, Bob, Edmund Burke, and Bill Pearl. *Getting in Shape.* Bolinas, CA: Shelter Publications, 1994.

Cooper, Kenneth H. *The Aerobics for Total Well-Being*. New York: Bantam Books, 1982.

Darden, Ellington. *Body Defining*. Chicago: NTC Contemporary Publishing Company, 1996.

Edwards, Diane and Kathy Nash. *Prime Moves*. Garden City Park, NY: Avery Publishing Group, 1992.

Pickney, Callan. *Callanetics*. New York: Avon Books, 1984.

EXERCISE PHYSIOLOGY, SPORTS MEDICINE

McArdle, William D., Frank I. Katch, and Victor L. Katch. *Exercise Physiology: Energy, Nutrition, and Human Performance*. Malvern, PA: Lea & Febiger, 1991.

Nieman, David C. *Fitness and Sports Medicine: A Health-Related Approach*. Palo Alto, CA: Bull Publishing Co., 1995.

Paffenbaiger, Jr. Ralph S., and Eric Olsen. *Life Fit*. Champaign, IL: Human Kinetics, 1996.

STRESS MANAGEMENT

Practical Guides

Borysenko, Joan. *Minding the Body, Mending the Mind*. New York: Bantam Books, 1987.

Charlesworth, Edward A. and Ronald G. Nathan. *Stress Management: A Comprehensive Guide to Wellness*. New York: Ballantine Books, 1985.

Davis, Martha, Elizabeth Robberins Eshelman, and Matthew McKay. *The Relaxation and Stress Reduction Workbook*. Oakland, CA: New Harbinger Publications, 1996.

Gawler, Ian. *Peace of Mind*. Garden City Park, NY: Avery Publishing Group, 1982.

Mason, L. John. *Guide to Stress Reduction*. Berkley, CA: Celestial Arts, 1985.

McKay, Matthew and Patrick Fanning. *Self-Esteem.* Oakland, CA: New Harbinger Publications, 1992.

Orioli, Esther M. and Robert K. Cooper. *Stressmap: The Ultimate Stress Management, Self-Assessment and Coping Guide Developed by Essi Systems.* New York: Newmarket Press, 1991.

Ornish, Dean. *Stress, Diet and Your Heart.* New York: Signet, 1982.

Powell, Trevor. *Free Yourself From Harmful Stress.* New York: DK Publishing, 1997.

Stress and Health Research

Cousins, Norman. *Anatomy of an Illness.* New York: Bantam Books, 1979.

Health. Pacific Grove, CA: Brooks/Cole Publishing Co., 1992.

Selye, Hans. *The Stress of Life.* Hightown, NJ: McGraw-Hill, Inc., 1984.

References

Allais, G., et al. "Patterns of Platelet Aggregation in Menstrual Migraine." *Cephalalgia*, Suppl 20 (Dec. 17, 1997):39–41.

Anthony, M. "Plasma Free Fatty Acids and Prostaglandin E1 in Migraine and Stress." *Headache* 16 (1976):58–63.

Anthony, M. "Role of Individual Free Fatty Acids in Migraine." *Res. Clin. Stud. Headache* 6 (1978):110–116.

Anthony, M., Lance, J.W. "The Possible Relationship of Serotonin to the Migraine Syndrome." *Res. Clin. Stud. Headache* 2 (1969):29–59.

Bic, Z., Blix, G.G., Hopp, H.P., Leslie, F.M. "In Search of the Ideal Treatment for Migraine Headache." *Medical Hypotheses* 50 (1998):1–7.

Bic, Z., et al. "The Influence of a Low-Fat Diet on Incidence and Severity of Migraine Headaches." *Journal of Women's Health & Gender-Based Medicine* 8 (5) (1999).

Blanchard, E.B., Andrasik, F. *Management of Chronic Headaches, a Psychological Approach.* New York: Pergamon Press Inc., 1985.

Carravalho, A.C., Colman, R.W., Lees, R.S. "Platelet Function in Hyperlipoproteinemia." *New England Journal of Medicine* 290 (1974):434.

Davidoff, R.A. *Migraine: Manifestations, Pathogenesis, and Management*. Philadelphia: F.A. Davis Company, 1995.

Hanington, E., Jones, R.J., Amess, J.A.L. "Platelet Aggregation in Response to 5-HT in Migraine Patients Taking Oral Contraceptives." *Lancet* (1982):967–968.

Leviton, A, Camenga, D. "Migraine Associated with Hyper-Pre-Beta Lipoproteinemia." *Neurology* 19 (1969).

McCarren, T. et al. "Amelioration of Severe Migraine by Fish Oil (omega-3) Fatty Acids." *Clinical Research* 32 (1985):275A.

Medina, J.L, Diamond, S. "The Role of Diet in Migraine." *Headache* 3 (1978):75–80.

Olesen, J., Tfelt-Hansen, P., Welch, K.M.A. *The Headaches*. New York: Raven Press Ltd., 1993.

Patterson, S.M., et al. "Effects of Acute Mental Stress on Serum Lipids: Mediating Effects of Plasma Volume." *Psychosomatic Medicine* 55(6) (Nov–Dec 1993):525–532.

Raskin, N.H. *Headache*. New York: Churchill Livingstone Inc., 1988.

Scrutton, M.C., Bawa, S. (1992). "5-HT, Platelets, and Migraine: Is There a Relationship?" *Frontiers in Headache Research*, Volume 2, edited by J. Olsen and P.R. Saxena. New York: Raven Press Ltd.

Widen, E., et al. "Insulin Resistance in Type 2 (non-insulin-dependent) Diabetic Patients with Hypertriglyceridemia." *Diabetologica* 35(12) (1992):1140–1145.

Yanagisawa, K. "The Effect of Body Fat Distribution on Glucose Tolerance in Overweight Subjects: Glucose Intolerance and Insulin Resistance Induced by Intra-Abdominal Fat Accumulation." *Folia Endocrinologica Japonica* 67(11) (Nov. 20, 1991): 1240–1251.

About the Authors

Zuzana Bic earned a doctorate in general medicine from King Charles University in Prague, Czech Republic in 1980. Her strong beliefs in prevention and lifestyle medicine led her to the School of Public Health at Loma Linda University, California, where she later earned her second doctorate in Public Health. She is currently working as an Assistant Adjunct Professor of Medicine at the University of California, Irvine, where she works with cancer patients and carries out research at the Chao Family Comprehensive Cancer Center. She also has a private office in Tustin, California, where she practices as a Preventive Care Specialist. Her approach is the application of integrated lifestyle medicine to the prevention and treatment of a variety of chronic diseases, including headaches.

L. Francis Bic holds a Ph.D. in Information and Computer Science. For the past twenty years, he has been a professor at the University of California, Irvine, where he teaches and carries out research in the area of biomedical computing. He is the author of several books and over 100 other scientific publications.

Index

Somatotropin, 71
Sports, active, 80
Stearic acid, 31. *See also* Blood fat.
Stress
    and body chemistry, 89–92
    chronic, 91–92
    headaches and, 36–37, 89–106. *See also* Headache triggers, lifestyle-related.
    guidelines for managing, 98–103
    identifying stressors, 101
    level of, categorizing, 100–101
    lifestyle modification approach to, 93–106
    occasional, 90–91
    response, 90
    techniques for managing. *See* Stress-management techniques.
Stress response, 90. *See also* Stress.
Stress-Management Technique Pyramid, 98–100
Stress-management techniques, 93–98
    assertiveness training, 98
    autogenics, 95
    biofeedback, 96
    coping skills, 97–98
    deep breathing, 94–95
    integrating with other activities, 101–103
    life-management skills, 98
    meditation, 96
    progressive muscle relaxation, 95
    relaxation techniques, 94–97
    self-hypnosis, 96–97
    visualization, 96
Stressors, 90, 92, 101. *See also* Stress.
Stretching exercises, 78. *See also* Physical activity, types of.
Strokes, lifestyle modification and, 13
Substance P, 13
Sucrose, 32–33, 48
Sumatriptan, 20
Supplemental approaches to treating headaches, 21. *See also* Alternative approaches to headache treatment; Minerals; Vitamins.
Systolic pressure, 112

Tension headaches, 10. *See also* Classification of headaches.
Theoretical Model of a Headache, 28, 29
Treatments for headaches
    alternative treatments, 20–22
    conventional treatments, 37–38
    lifestyle modification approach, 2, 3, 8, 22–24
    over-the-counter medications, 18–19
    prescription medications, 19–20
Trepanation, 11, 14
Triglycerides, 31. *See also* Blood fat.
Tryptophan, 30, 50, 52
Tylenol, 18
Type II diabetes, lifestyle modification and, 12–13. *See also* Disease, chronic, lifestyle factors and.
Tyramine, 27, 52, 53. *See also* Headache triggers, chemical.

Uncontrollable stressors, 101
United States Department of Agriculture (USDA), 56, 59

Vasoconstriction, 28
Vasodilatation, 28, 30, 35, 36
Vegetables, increasing intake of, 59
Visualization, 96. *See also* Relaxation techniques; Stress-management techniques.
Vitamin A, 52
Vitamin B_2 (riboflavin), 52
Vitamin B_3 (niacin), 52
Vitamin B_6 (pyridoxine) and serotonin levels, 30, 52
Vitamin C, 52
Vitamins, 21, 52. *See also* individual vitamins.

Water, 51
    increasing intake of, 61–62
White blood cells, 31. *See also* Blood, makeup of.
Whole-grain products, increasing intake of, 58
Willow bark *(Salicis cortex)*, 21
World Health Organization, 8